NLP and Coaching for Health Professionals

C000175304

NLP and Coaching for Healthcare Professionals:

Developing Expert Practice

Authors

SUZANNE HENWOOD

JIM LISTER

Contributor: Liz Holland

John Wiley & Sons, Ltd

Copyright © 2007   John Wiley & Sons, Ltd
The Atrium, Southern Gate, Chichester,
West Sussex PO19 8SQ, England
Telephone   (+44) 1243 779777

Email (for orders and customer service enquiries): cs-books@wiley.co.uk
Visit our Home Page on www.wiley.com

All Rights Reserved. No part of this publication may be reproduced, stored in a retrieval system or
transmitted in any form or by any means, electronic, mechanical, photocopying, recording, scanning or
otherwise, except under the terms of the Copyright, Designs and Patents Act 1988 or under the terms of a
licence issued by the Copyright Licensing Agency Ltd, 90 Tottenham Court Road, London W1T 4LP, UK,
without the permission in writing of the Publisher. Requests to the Publisher should be addressed to the
Permissions Department, John Wiley & Sons Ltd, The Atrium, Southern Gate, Chichester, West Sussex
PO19 8SQ, England, or emailed to permreq@wiley.co.uk, or faxed to (+44) 1243 770620.

Designations used by companies to distinguish their products are often claimed as trademarks. All brand
names and product names used in this book are trade names, service marks, trademarks or registered
trademarks of their respective owners. The Publisher is not associated with any product or vendor
mentioned in this book.

This publication is designed to provide accurate and authoritative information in regard to the subject
matter covered. It is sold on the understanding that the Publisher is not engaged in rendering professional
services. If professional advice or other expert assistance is required, the services of a competent
professional should be sought.

Other Wiley Editorial Offices

John Wiley & Sons Inc., 111 River Street, Hoboken, NJ 07030, USA

Jossey-Bass, 989 Market Street, San Francisco, CA 94103-1741, USA

Wiley-VCH Verlag GmbH, Boschstr. 12, D-69469 Weinheim, Germany

John Wiley & Sons Australia Ltd, 42 McDougall Street, Milton, Queensland 4064, Australia

John Wiley & Sons (Asia) Pte Ltd, 2 Clementi Loop #02-01, Jin Xing Distripark, Singapore 129809

John Wiley & Sons Canada Ltd, 6045 Freemont Blvd, Mississauga, ONT, L5R 4J3

Wiley also publishes its books in a variety of electronic formats. Some content that appears in print may
not be available in electronic books.

Anniversary Logo Design: Richard J. Pacifico

Library of Congress Cataloging-in-Publication Data

Henwood, Suzanne.
    NLP and coaching for healthcare professionals : developing expert practice / written by
Suzanne Henwood, Jim Lister ; contribution by Liz Holland.
        p. ; cm.
    Includes bibliographical references and index.
    ISBN-13: 978-0-470-06573-0 (pbk. : alk. paper)
    ISBN-10: 0-470-006573-7 (pbk. : alk. paper)
    1. Medical personnel – Mental health.   2. Neurolinguistic programming.   I. Lister, Jim.
II. Holland, Liz.   III. Title.   IV. Title: Neurolinguistic programming and coaching for
healthcare professionals.
    [DNLM: 1. Health Personnel.   2. Neurolinguistic Programming.   3. Communication.
4. Goals.   5. Self Concept.   6. Staff Development – methods.
W 21 H528n 2007]
    RC451.4.M44H46 2007
    610.69 – dc22
                                                                                    2006036940

A catalogue record for this book is available from the British Library
ISBN 13: 978-0-470-06573-0

Typeset by SNP Best-set Typesetter Ltd., Hong Kong
Printed and bound in Great Britain by TJ International Ltd, Padstow, Cornwall

This book is printed on acid-free paper responsibly manufactured from sustainable forestry in which at
least two trees are planted for each one used for paper production.

Dedication

We dedicate this book to our next generation. Who knows, maybe they too will move into the healthcare professions, maybe not. We hope that whatever they do they will do it excellently, enjoying every minute of finding their full potential and living out their dreams:

Rebekah, Benjamin and Barney, and Rohanna

Suzanne Henwood

Jim Lister

Contents

About the authors and contributor

Authors

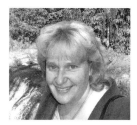

Suzanne Henwood

Suzanne is a Master Practitioner in both NLP and Time Line Therapy and holds a doctorate in CPD Effectiveness and an MSc in Applied Radiography. She runs her own business in coaching and training and works to develop services through people development, through a strong belief in the need to invest in and support people so that they can fulfil their potentials and improve services provided.

Suzanne is a radiographer by professional background and spent many years in education, finishing her university career as Director of Postgraduate Studies in Health at a London university. From there she moved to a large UK charity, where she managed a National Institute of Education, based in seven universities around the country, providing leading edge education and development initiatives to a range of professional disciplines in the field of cancer and palliative care.

In 2005 she set up her own company, with a number of associates, taking NLP into the healthcare community in order to influence and change practice, through individual professionals and the teams in which they work.

Suzanne holds an adjunct professorship in Auckland, New Zealand and sits on a Department of Health advisory group for strategy and policy in health and social care. She works at professional body level for the College and Society of Radiographers and continues to be passionate about improving services for patients and staff alike.

Contact: henwoodassociates@btinternet.com

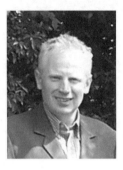

Jim Lister

Jim Lister is a Master Practitioner in NLP and has worked as a trainer and coach within his own business, the C:Change Partnership, for the past nine years. Jim's work is spread over the private, public and charitable sectors, and has developed a focus around designing work within healthcare settings.

Over the past three years, Jim has been employed extensively by Macmillan Cancer Support, and has delivered a lecture programme to postholders exploring many of the themes contained within this book. He also works with NHS Trusts in both South and North Wales to help build effective teams and develop individuals.

He works alongside Suzanne in delivering short programmes of change for the College and Society of Radiographers. He is also working for the National Association of Complementary Therapists supporting staff employed in hospices throughout the UK.

Contact: jimlister@cchangepartnership.co.uk

Contributor

Liz Holland

Liz has more than 30 years' experience in radiology having originally qualified as a Medical Radiation Technologist before moving into management of the radiology services at Dunedin Hospital, New Zealand. She left radiology to work in health-related change management projects where she experienced the impact of having her position made redundant. She left the health sector and developed a 'portfolio' career being employed part time as a career consultant with Career Services and establishing her private business as a professional supervisor and Life Coach. Liz qualified as a Life Coach through the virtual university, Coach U. She now works with a wide range of people of different ages, ethnicity, educational and health backgrounds, assisting them to clarify how they want to live their lives.

Liz also offers custom-designed workshops to assist workplaces or groups with an issue or goal they wish to achieve.

She is a member of the International Coach Federation, Career Practitioners Association of New Zealand and the NZ Institute of Medical Radiation Technologists. She holds a Diploma of the College of Radiographers (London); NZOQ Certificate in Quality Assurance and is the recipient of an Honorary Masters degree in Health Science (Medical Radiation Technology) from Unitec New Zealand.

Contact: lizholland@xtra.co.nz

Foreword

Jeremy Lazarus

It's an honour to be asked to write the foreword for *NLP and Coaching for Healthcare Professionals: Developing Expert Practice.*

When I first met Suzanne in July 2005 on one of my Introduction to NLP courses, she was, shall we say, cynical about the usefulness to her and others of NLP. Here we are, a little over 18 months later, and Suzanne is co-authoring a book on the uses of NLP in the healthcare sector, a subject which is dear to my heart. What a turnaround! It was a privilege to train her and witness this change of heart and attitude.

In this book the authors cover the uses of NLP and related topics in the context of how to improve levels of effectiveness in dealings with other people, be they colleagues, staff, bosses or patients. The topics covered also have benefits for improving readers' communication with friends and family, as well as benefits for readers' own self-development.

For some, the main interest in reading this book will be on making work communication and results even better than they currently are. At the other end of the spectrum, some readers will be starting from a rather dissatisfied position at work and be looking for ways to make more significant and urgent changes in their role and with their teams. Wherever you are on the spectrum, the techniques and tips provided in *NLP and Coaching for Healthcare Professionals* will help guide you, and help you guide others, to make some of the changes that you require.

In terms of NLP itself, the book outlines its meaning and underlying concepts. The reason for my particular interest and passion for NLP is quite simple – it works! As a former accountant, finance director and management consultant, I am only interested in tools and techniques for use in a business and work environment if they produce results. NLP fits the bill perfectly. In addition, having trained several medical professionals in NLP, including neurosurgeons, GPs, nurses, radiographers and administrative staff, they are as enthusiastic as I am about its usefulness and applicability to the medical world.

So, whatever your particular role within the healthcare sector, and wherever you are in terms of your satisfaction with your current situation within it, take as much as you can from this book for yourself and those who you believe and feel would benefit from it.

Enjoy!

Jeremy Lazarus
Director, The Lazarus Consultancy Ltd
Certified Trainer of NLP

- no. of pt's per day
  - (A) v 2 c. admin ? lunch week.

- (I get inpatient)

- writing as I listen
  - (A) after i notes

- unable to Book pt :- as free.
  - (A) Block

- taking card details
  - (A) ask pt to CBO

vater, bracknell, m4).

30am)

ee named above and may contain confidential or legally privileged information. If you a
disseminate to other parties or otherwise use the contents of this email. It is the respons
might affect any computer or IT system into which they are received and opened. NUFF
il and any attachments Nuffield Health: Nuffield Health Registered Office: Epsom Gatew
arity Registered in Scotland Number: SC041793 and a Company Limited by Guarantee

Preface

Lisa Wake

I seem to have spent most of my adult life in some form of relationship with the NHS. My early childhood had a strong influence on my chosen career as a nurse, and full of enthusiasm to be a modern Florence Nightingale I entered nursing at the tender age of 18. This enthusiasm for the caring profession stayed with me for about 10 years, but I became increasingly frustrated with the 'stuckness' of the system in which I worked and eventually I decided to swap sides. I became a manager, again enthusiastic about how I could make a difference to the system, this time by managing it, rather than just working within it. After another five years, during which time I met NLP as a methodology of performance excellence, I decided to use this newfound skill base to pursue a career supporting the NHS and other systems from the outside. I remain attached to the NHS through both my clinical role as a psychotherapist and my training and consultancy work.

I can clearly recall the first time I met this 'thing' called NLP. A colleague was supporting me to find new ways to manage my manager. I had developed a strategy of listening to the footsteps of my manager as they came down the corridor and would then decide to pick up the phone and pretend to be busy, so that I could avoid the ire that would inevitably follow. Although a tactic that created delay, it did not address the underlying relationship difficulty that I was having. My colleague helped me to identify more useful ways of handling this relationship; even something as simple as standing up when my manager was about to march into my office seemed to diffuse the situation somewhat.

Suzanne, Jim and Liz have brought together some of the very simple tools and techniques that exist within NLP to enable you to make a difference to your own effectiveness and the effectiveness of others. Fired by their enthusiasm for their subject and passion for the NHS, all three of them offer a clear understanding of NLP and its direct application to your work. This book provides very concrete examples of how major differences can be made to working lives through some very small interventions.

I am delighted to recommend this book to you and hope that you will find within it some useful advice, ideas or tools that will enable you to continue and extend your work with patients, clients and service users.

Lisa Wake
UKCP Registered Neurolinguistic Psychotherapist
INLPTA Certified Trainer of NLP

Acknowledgements

We have so many people to thank it is difficult to know who to include here. We have to start by thanking our partners, who have encouraged, supported, helped, inspired and generally kept the family going while we have dedicated our time to this book. So thank you to Phil and Katherine.

We also want to say thank you to those people who introduced us to NLP, to Sheila Young and Nicci Evans. To those who trained us so superbly; Jeremy Lazarus, John Seymour and Lisa Wake; their passion for NLP was infectious and not only did they train us, they have also helped deepen our understanding of NLP and how to use it ethically and to a very high standard. We will always be indebted to them for that. Through these great people we found a new way of living, and they also continue to support and inspire us as we carry on our journey of learning and discovery and as we grow ourselves.

Thank you too to Liz Holland for contributing her wider coaching knowledge and expertise. Her enthusiasm and attention to detail hugely enhanced this book.

To the Lister family and especially Rob Lister for his patience and attention to detail.

To all those who have helped contribute to the development of the C:Change Partnership, especially Kay Douglas, Sonja Martin and all colleagues and staff at CRL especially Mark Leonard, Kevin Lee and David Large.

To Pawel Abbott, Rob Edwards and especially to Danny Schofield for being open to new ideas and making them work, despite the doubters.

To the team at Wiley for believing in our vision and for supporting us through to publication.

Finally to all our clients, who allow us to walk with them on their journeys, and especially those who allowed us to share their stories through this book. You have our lasting gratitude.

Introduction

Suzanne Henwood

1

> Don't be frightened to dream dreams – it is by dreaming that you start to become what you want to become

As busy healthcare practitioners, I imagine you are already over-committed with work, CPD and other responsibilities, so why should you take valuable time out to read this book? Well, we believe this is probably one of the most important books you will ever read on developing excellence in healthcare practice, through developing yourself. This is a book to inspire and motivate you, to increase your self-awareness and to empower you so that you can be whatever it is you want to be. It is about recognising the potential within you and empowering you so that you may thrive and be a respected expert practitioner and leader in your field. It is our belief that by focusing on you and your internal development, you will achieve far more than in many other CPD activities, which are focused on a specific ability or competence to practise in a particular clinical area. This book is different; it will change you at your very core – if you want it to. It will help you to find out who you are and where you are going. This book is an investment in you.

Whether you are currently thriving in your career, getting by, or struggling to go to work every day, whether you work in a supportive and learning environment, or whether you are working in a more negative environment where there is little regard for your own development and where you do not feel valued, this book can take you to the next level on your own personal and career pathway. Whether you have just qualified, or whether you are close to retirement, this book is equally relevant to you.

Walt Disney is famously quoted as saying 'If you can dream it, you can do it'. What do you dream? What is it you want to achieve? What in the past has been holding you back? If you read this book dreaming your dreams and openly and honestly engaging with the tools and techniques we outline, you will change, you will grow, and our hope is that you will find renewed passion in your profession, compassion for your patients and you will hugely increase your ability to achieve and be successful.

Are you ready to start a journey that could change the way you think? This book will give you the tools to help you thrive within change. It will give you the ability to recharge your batteries as and when they need recharging, and it will give you renewed focus and energy. You will learn more about yourself so that you can give even more of yourself at work (and at home). We have been so impressed with the impact of the tools in our own work and lives that we had to share them with you. When you have your own stories of change to tell, get in touch – we would love to hear how this book helped you.

Why are we so passionate about sharing this material with you? As a healthcare practitioner myself, I know how stressful the healthcare environment can be. I understand the pressures that have to be faced by individual practitioners and health service departments. I have seen and worked in some of the difficult cultures that exist within healthcare, as well as being privileged to have worked in wonderfully supportive and inspiring departments, where I knew exactly why I had become a healthcare professional. Now I want to do what I can to help practitioners realise their full potential and be the very best they can be, regardless of where they are working. The tools in this book can be an enormous help both to those who are struggling and those who are thriving. I hope that in helping individuals we can, little by little, work together to continually improve the services we provide. By reading this book, I hope you too become inspired afresh; and that through your own journey you will also get excited again about the power you have as an individual to make a difference and to influence change. Through a philosophy of respect and a deep desire to care for patients, I hope that together, in small stages, we can model professional pride in being a healthcare practitioner. I hope that you take the things you learn from this book and share them. I hope that you find renewed enthusiasm for caring and providing for patients in new and innovative ways by finding your own power within. This is the vision that I share with you. Even now I hope you are feeling excited, that you are already thinking of all the things you want to do to make a difference, all the things you want to achieve; even now let yourself feel how good that is going to feel – feel and imagine what it is going to be like to do the job you love, in the way that you want, where you know you are making a real difference. Maybe you are lucky enough to be in that position already. If this is not yet reality for you and this is a vision that you have for yourself, then read on and I, along with my co-authors, will show you how to move things forward so that your vision becomes your reality. It would be a privilege to share some of that journey with you through the pages of this book.

About the book

This book is designed as a tool kit to enable you to increase your own self-awareness in order to allow you to achieve self-empowerment – skills that are fundamental to leadership at any level, but also we believe essential to all health-care practitioners. The book is designed to give you tools that you can use to increase your flexibility in an ever-changing environment, to allow you to thrive within periods of change. It is a book which focuses on you, your needs and your values, as it is our belief that change has to start within. It is through personal change that we will have the maximum impact on the environment we work in.

You can read the book from front to back, and that might be a useful start to give yourself an initial overview of what it can offer, to begin to inspire you and excite you about the possibilities for further development. Each tool can then be used and applied to your own needs and can be used at your own pace. You can select which tool you want to use to reflect where you are on your own journey or to respond to a particular issue of concern you are currently facing. Each tool is flexible and can be used time and time again in different contexts, so you can refer back to it regularly and re-use it, each time moving further on and revealing deeper and deeper layers about yourself. Many of the tools are available on the website referred to later in this chapter.

The chapters are written by three very different people, with very different backgrounds, professionally and geographically, though we all now work as coaches and/or trainers offering services to healthcare practitioners, many of whom have contributed their stories to this book to give you a real sense of where the tools have already been successfully used in healthcare practice. While we have aimed to bring the style of the book into one cohesive whole, we have allowed the individuality of each author to remain, giving you even greater access to a variety of approaches and perspectives on this important subject. We have all contributed to all of the chapters, the name on any one chapter represents the person who led that chapter; the material within has been developed and refined by each of us to give it even greater potential impact.

The key to this book, as we have already said, is a focus on self. Change starts internally. It is through internal change that we see external changes in behaviour and in our impact on others. If we get that focus wrong, we will not be as successful and nothing will really change.

There is a wonderful story I have often heard told and which I have re-written here in the context of modern day healthcare. It is the story of two nurses from the same ward both of whom have been qualified for two years and are looking to move to new jobs. They hear about an excellent coach and decide to approach this person to obtain advice on changing jobs:

Nurse 1: 'So, as I said, I am thinking of moving to the hospital in the neighbouring Trust. Do you know of it?'
Coach: 'I do'.
Nurse 1: 'Can you tell me what it is like?'
Coach: 'What is the hospital like that you are thinking of leaving?'
Nurse 1: 'It isn't very nice. The staff are not friendly, I am not well supported and I never seem to fit in.'
Coach: 'You will find the hospital in the neighbouring Trust very similar.'
The first nurse left the session confused. She had been looking for direction.
The second nurse booked an appointment with the same coach.

Nurse 2: 'So, as I said, I am thinking of moving to the hospital in the neighbouring Trust. Do you know of it?'
Coach: 'I do'.
Nurse 2: 'Can you tell me what it is like?'
Coach: 'What is the hospital like that you are thinking of leaving?'
Nurse 2: 'It's great. I get on really well with the staff, I am challenged and have learnt a great deal.'
Coach: 'You will find the hospital in the neighbouring Trust very similar.'

If there is one key lesson to learn in this book it is get to know yourself completely and then change aspects in you that are not producing the results you want. You will be surprised how quickly things around you change once you have made that sincere change within yourself. You will see things differently and people will see you differently, and consequently everything changes. How great will you feel when you have made the changes you want and start to get the results you want?

So, we urge you to go on. Give yourself the time and scope you need to make this work for you. Treat yourself to some real devotional time and get to know who you are. We guarantee that it will be time well spent and you will benefit both personally and professionally.

It is worth saying what the book is not. It is not a theoretical text and does not spend a great deal of time looking at either the history or development of the tools we describe, or indeed at the evidence for their effectiveness. Texts to establish the history and credibility of NLP already exist. We do, however, offer at the end of the book a recommended reading list, which offers some of our favourite books on the subjects raised here. If it suits your own way of learning and you like to see evidence of the potential benefit of new techniques some or all of these books may help you to understand the tools more deeply and see for yourself how you could apply them in practice. And it may be that as you work through the tools and experience change within yourself, you will be happy to use them as we present them here. Maybe even now you are thinking about how you learn and about how you might use these tools in your practice. Do whatever it takes for you to use this material effectively. This 'how to,' if you like, of using NLP and other coaching techniques is offered to you as a healthcare practitioner, with the hope that you use the skills to the full in your professional practice and in your personal life.

Having said what the book is not, let us explain why we believe it is essential reading for healthcare practitioners. It is our belief that if the contents of this book are applied in practice they will have a huge impact on you as a person, both within your own personal life and in your professional practice. It provides tools which can be used in practice to manage difficult situations and to enable you to get the results you want. It also provides a framework to reflect on your own practice, which is frequently a requirement of CPD programmes.

Perhaps it would be worth you spending a few moments, before you start reading the book fully, just thinking about what it is you want to get out of the book, what your needs are, what it is you hope to learn for you. Just make a note of what it is you want in your own development; what it was that made you pick up this book. What would make this the best book on personal and professional development you have ever read?

What would make this the best personal and professional development book I have ever read?

Now you have looked specifically at what you hope to gain from the book, let us outline for you what we believe it will offer.

The book starts by introducing you to the concepts of NLP and coaching. While NLP techniques are not the only tools described in the book, they form a large part of it, and we want to share with you briefly where NLP came from and the power that it offers. We also explore some of the wider aspects of coaching, and we are delighted to have alongside us a qualified and experienced coach from New Zealand, Liz Holland, who has more than 35 years' experience in the health sector as a practitioner, manager and influencer at government level. Liz will help us to introduce the benefits of coaching in healthcare, and will explain some of the 'Coach U' tools and techniques to complement the NLP techniques that Jim and I will explain. We will introduce the importance of the mind-body link and some of the potential benefits to you in pursuing this material, taking you way beyond just professional development and expert practice.

NLP and coaching can have a beneficial impact on your health and well-being too, by giving you a sense of inner strength, peace, satisfaction and congruence (or being aligned inside), which leads to renewed motivation to fulfil your purpose in life. We will introduce to you the concept of timing and why there is no better time than now to begin your journey with us.

You will see that throughout the book we bring you real-life examples of where the tools and techniques have been used in practice. In order to retain the anonymity of our clients, we have changed all the names, and in some cases the gender, and removed any indication of workplace location. They know who they are and we value their contribution to this book. Thank you. We are continually grateful that our clients are willing to share their journeys with us, and through their openness and active participation allow us to keep growing ourselves. It is a privilege and a pleasure to share with you all.

In Chapter 2 we focus on self-empowerment, discussing the importance of the mind-body link. We look at our 'internal dialogue' that is used to affect our attitude and our behaviour and consequently our results. We look at how we all create internal representations of reality and how that determines how we feel and act in response. We describe some powerful tools which enable us to look at our own internal linguistics and explore some practical steps on how to change how we feel internally, thus taking the first step towards outward change.

Chapter 3 looks at how we empower ourselves to others. Building on Chapter 2, it looks at how our own awareness can be enhanced so that we can adapt our internal representations to give a more positive image of any given situation. We explore well-known concepts such as body language and building rapport, to a level we had never encountered in healthcare practitioner training before. We look briefly at examples of advanced use of language, and at body language cues that can literally transform how we interact with both patients and colleagues, thus revolutionising our practice.

In Chapter 4 we begin to look at how to take this new knowledge and move forward with it in the direction we want to travel. We look at a tool to help assess whether or not all aspects of our lives are in balance, an essential skill if we are to remain productive and effective in our careers. We reinforce the need to take care of 'self' in order to continue caring for others.

Chapter 5 begins to explore how this new increased self-awareness links to our depth of knowledge about our own departments or organisations. The chapter explores the issue of personal and corporate values, and introduces a tool to assess how well we 'fit' and consequently how we can contribute even more effectively at work by adapting what we do to correspond to the mission and values in the workplace.

In Chapter 6 we introduce an incredibly powerful tool that has numerous applications. One of its common uses is within conflict resolution, but it can also be used to look at new directions, strategy building, decision making, enabling two teams to work together more effectively, or exploring personal reactions to particular issues from different perspectives. Once you have mastered this tool you will find that it can be easily adapted so that it can be introduced seamlessly into meetings without colleagues realising you are using a tool at all.

In Chapter 7 we begin to bring together what you have learned so far and help you set goals to ensure you start to realise your dreams. With clear goals and with a real focus it is much more likely that you will begin to achieve something spectacular. In order to achieve what you dream of you need to know where you want to move to, and you need to know what you must do to achieve that outcome. This tool is an excellent way to commit yourself to making the changes required so that you get the results you want.

Chapter 8 follows up the writing of goals with a set of tools forming a self-management tool kit. This chapter is jam-packed with practical tools to empower and enthuse you to make sure that you pursue your dreams. After implementing these techniques you will have no excuse for not making your dreams come true! The concept of 'time lines' will enable you to determine when exactly you will achieve your desired outcomes. We will show you how to make your goals so compelling that you will be keen to finish the book so you can get on with making things happen!

Chapter 9 recognises the reality of busy lives and looks at ways to ensure you retain your initial enthusiasm and keep your momentum going, while you also care for yourself effectively. It is unlikely you will need to refer back to this chapter very often as you are going to be striving ahead to reach your goals; it might then be more useful to share with colleagues who have only just begun their journeys.

In Chapter 10 we conclude by briefly drawing all your learning together and by emphasising just how far you have already come by having finished the book. We will give you some tips on finding a coach, in particular how to ensure that a coach is credible and suitably qualified. We will reinforce how you are central to this whole process and especially central to its success. You can achieve anything you put your mind to, if you know what it is you wish to achieve and if you believe in yourself. The fact you are reading this is a phenomenal starting point. We believe you can achieve more than you ever dreamed possible. We believe you are aspiring leaders in your field who really make a difference in healthcare and who could do even more. If you have any doubts, find a coach and work through those doubts. Nothing and no one can hold you back from achieving your dreams, except you. If you feel blocked, if you don't believe in your own ability to achieve your dreams, you need to find a way to change, and there are ways to change.

We are really excited about sharing this material with you because each one of us has experienced for ourselves the power of the tools we describe. We have all started on a journey to greater self-awareness that has hugely transformed who we are and what we can achieve. We know this is possible for you as well and we look forward to hearing from you about how this book has literally changed the way you think and the way you work, through changing the way you feel, the way you behave and the results you get for you and your patients. Allow yourself to get excited. Allow yourself to dream. You have already begun the most exciting journey there is. Enjoy the ride.

In order to offer you additional support, we have also set up a website www.wiley.com/go/nlphealthcare where you will find copies of many of the tools from within this book to enable you to use them over and over again. For access to this website you will require the unique code indicated on the site. You can also contact us through the website or directly if you want additional individual support on your own journey, and we would love to hear from you regarding your experience of using these tools in practice; and share your successes and dreams. Our contact details are on pp. ix, x and xi. We look forward to hearing from you.

So what is NLP?

It is difficult to say categorically what NLP is. There are numerous definitions available, each offering a slightly different perspective and focus, and view of exactly what it can achieve. If we break NLP into its three main components we can see that 'neuro' relates to neurology. Neurology in medical terminology is the study of the nervous system and its diseases. In NLP it is the study of the mind and brain and in particular how we think about things and how we process information. We experience life through our five senses and internally we process that information and behave accordingly. This places NLP at the core of who we are; it is about what we think inside, how we interpret our reality. NLP will probably challenge your view of the world and open new doors to allow you to see other points of view and to explore other perspectives. NLP will also enable you to see how closely the mind and body work together, and how by changing one you can create a huge impact on the other.

'Linguistic' is all about language skills. In NLP terms this is how we use language to communicate and how other people's use of language affects us. It includes how we use language to structure our thoughts and to communicate those thoughts to others. In NLP what you say is important, and how you say it and what you mean by it is even more important.

'Programming' refers to how we plan how to react (not always consciously) to achieve specific goals. It is how we organise and store our ideas (and our actions). This is probably the most controversial aspect of NLP as some people feel it implies some form of manipulation. Once you get to understand the philosophy behind NLP you will see just how far from the truth this is. NLP is about respecting each individual's values and beliefs and working with those values to achieve great results, whilst considering the impact of any changes on other people. If you doubt whether you are naturally programmed in any way, consider what happens when you hear a fire alarm, when you hear a resuscitation bleep go off or when you hear someone say something to you which generates a particular response in you. Many of our behaviours are learned and we are programmed throughout life to react to certain stimuli in a certain way. NLP allows us to identify some of that programming which is unhelpful, which has happened subconsciously, and decide on whether or not it is a behavioural programme we wish to maintain. NLP also allows us to programme new behaviours to get the results we want; it establishes choice within our own programming and gives us control.

To bring this together then, NLP is the study and practice of how we think, how we use language to communicate, and how we develop ways to react to external and internal stimuli, thus generating behaviours which determine our actions. It gives a depth of understanding about ourselves that allows us to strive towards and achieve excellence in practice; this is essential when we use any element of leadership skills, and when looking at how to be more effective. As if that were not enough, NLP not only changes the way we think, talk and act, thus enabling us to transform ourselves into being truly expert professional practitioners, it also impacts on our self image so that we learn to love, respect and care for ourselves, so allowing us to live life to the full.

Some of the published definitions include:

- NLP is the art and science of personal excellence (O'Connor and Seymour, 1990).

- NLP is the study of what works in thinking, language and behaviour. It is a way of coding and reproducing excellence that enables you to consistently achieve the results that you want both for yourself, for your business and for your life (Knight, 2002).
- NLP is the influence of language on our mind and subsequent behaviour (O'Connor, 2001).

NLP started in the 1970s when two academics in California, John Grinder and Richard Bandler, began to work together looking at the effectiveness of three highly regarded therapists. They spent hours watching and modelling the successful practice of the three therapists and identified some common patterns, from which they developed a model, or set of tools, which could be used to enhance communication, to accelerate learning and personal understanding, and to effect real and lasting change.

Over time the tools of NLP have been further refined and developed, and they continue to evolve so that they can be applied across many contexts. Talk to anyone who has been coached or trained using NLP techniques, and you will hear of excellence and powerful personal transformation. We describe some of those tools in this book to bring NLP into healthcare practice, alongside other coaching techniques which we have personally used and approved in practice.

Why is NLP and coaching relevant to healthcare today?

Within healthcare we are living in a world of constant change. We are no longer secure in our once familiar environments and instead face constant uncertainty. The healthcare environment is rapidly progressing and becoming more and more complex. Roles are extending and new roles are being developed. We are being constantly challenged to remain up to date and to develop new skills and competences. The rate of change is also increasing, making it more and more difficult to keep up.

Healthcare practitioners therefore need new skills to cope in this new world. Their initial training, supplemented by traditional forms of CPD is no longer enough. They need to be able to have a central core of calm and control in order to be able to practise effectively. They need to be able to take care of themselves, so that they in turn can care for others.

As healthcare practitioners you need to be able to respond to change and yet also have the expertise to retain what works well. You need advanced communication skills in order to ensure that your patients are comfortable and informed within a potentially chaotic healthcare environment and to encourage patients to become active care partners instead of passive recipients of care. You also need to be able to communicate at an advanced level with other healthcare practitioners who are facing different, yet equally disturbing changes, and who might also feel insecure and threatened. And, finally, you need to be able to communicate internally with yourselves to make sense of your values, beliefs, feelings and reactions, to truly reflect on your practice. In the midst of any such radical and fast-paced change there will be differences of opinion. Future expert practitioners, using tools like those we present here, will be able to appreciate others' points of view and to discuss and negotiate so that practice is continually developed, thereby reducing potential conflict or unnecessary stress.

Why is NLP and coaching so relevant to healthcare? We would go further and say it is essential. Without it healthcare practitioners may struggle to cope with the pace and scope of change in the future. With NLP you will have the ability, not only to cope with the changes, but also to actively influence and direct those changes. You will enjoy and be passionate about your practice as you fulfil and live out your values, enacting your beliefs about making a real difference for your patients. You will thrive on the challenges, and you will work together with other colleagues to make improvements. You will build up and leave behind you a legacy of expert practice for others to follow.

You might be wondering where coaching fits in relation to other initiatives, for example, mentoring, clinical supervision, preceptorship and even appraisal and development planning. In brief, mentoring is likely to be a longer-term relationship and is usually done by a more experienced practitioner from the same field of practice, for example, for someone needing support early on in any aspect of career change. Clinical supervision is a varied term adopted by some professions. Again it can be undertaken by a more senior or experienced practitioner in the same field who helps to problem solve and to increase understanding of particular issues, or it can be very close to coaching, in which someone gets alongside a practitioner for a period of time and helps them to truly reflect on their own practice. Preceptorship tends to be a more formalised approach to assist and support someone who is changing roles. Alternatively, when employees enter clinical practice, preceptorship can be a time to offer guidance before expecting them to work completely autonomously. It is our belief that coaching sits comfortably alongside these other practices. Coaching is effective in its own right as a form of personal and professional development and in addition it will allow individuals to be effective in each of the other related areas, for example to prepare fully for appraisal and development planning and to know how to get the most out of a mentoring or supervisory relationship.

There is much to be said for considering using an external coach who is separate from any organisational obligation, so that you can discuss fully and openly any aspect of your practice. Indeed for the foreseeable future it is likely that there will not be sufficient numbers of trained coaches dedicated to the healthcare sector. Having said that, the tools can be used 'by self for self' and can also be used in a peer coaching relationship where two professionals decide to support each other by using the tools together. Each individual would just have to assess any potential conflict of interest, or ethical issues that might arise as a result of sharing at such depth. Over time peers might wish to seek external coaching to gain full benefit from the complete range of tools and techniques available. A unique aspect of some of the tools outlined in this book is that they can be used 'content free' so that case details do not have to be disclosed, which opens up the scope for who they can be undertaken with.

What can NLP offer?

NLP is valuable in so many contexts. It is effective for both personal and professional development. We outline here just some of the most important benefits for healthcare practitioners:

- By using NLP you will learn to communicate more effectively. Within healthcare the skill of effective communication is vital. What impact does your comment have on a patient when you say, 'Oh yes you have osteoporosis, this is where the bones crumble,' or when you say to someone, 'It is very easy to get depressed in this situation'. We need to seriously start to question the terminology we use which might generate negative internal representations in our patients, a process which might have an undesirable impact on their potential health and/or recovery. This is in addition to all the communication which occurs between colleagues and teams which can often be combative and excessively competitive, rather than empowering and encouraging, not to mention our own internal communication, which often works to restrict and criticise us, instead of being used to encourage and build us up.

- In terms of CPD, NLP could be the most effective personal and professional development you have ever undertaken. If you determine effectiveness by its ability to impact on your practice and its ability to improve the services you offer, NLP will do both of those things, naturally and easily, without you even really focusing on that as an outcome.

- NLP will blow your map of the world. You will change the way you think and you will know and respect yourself in a new and exciting way. If you remain unsure about this, you would gain hugely from finding yourself a reputable coach who can work through some of the more personal aspects of your development, which may be holding you back in your professional practice. Some of these things might include your own self-esteem, your confidence, and your belief in your ability to be an expert practitioner or leader in your field. Once you have sorted these issues out, you will feel and behave like a new person.

- Finally, NLP is at the very heart of leadership excellence. NLP enables you not only to understand yourself fully, but also to understand your colleagues and staff so that you can enable them to work to their strengths and acknowledge safely the areas that still require development.

Some of the key guiding principles of NLP include:

- People respond to their own experience, not to reality itself. If you can enhance their experience by encouraging and nurturing them, you could change a person's reality and transform them into a motivated, confident practitioner who works hard and effectively in the team.
- People make the best choice they can at the time. If you take this on board as a guiding principle, there is no blame in making mistakes, and you can generate a genuine learning culture where individuals can grow and develop.
- Every behaviour has a positive intention. By looking at what that positive intention is in any given situation you can look at a difficult context in a completely different way.
- The meaning of any communication is the response you get. By taking full responsibility for the effectiveness of your own communication you will transform the communication in your team by ensuring that what others heard and understood is actually what you meant to say.
- We have, or can obtain, all the resources we need to do the job expertly. Exploring with staff what skills and abilities they have, and then helping them to fill any gaps, will hugely release staff to work better and even more effectively, whilst also showing they are valued and trusted to keep developing.

You can see how this impacts not only on leadership but also on management. If you are still unsure what the difference between the two is, leadership sets the direction that people choose to follow, and management steers the team in that direction, making sure the team keep on track. Put another way:

> 'In a changing environment, a manager will work to understand the individuals in his or her team, adapting to their needs and helping them to cope with change. Like a shepherd, the manager's goal is to get the team to achieve the objective. A leader is more interested in the goal itself and providing a vision of that goal that is inspiring. A leader requires followers to commit to the cause, to choose to follow and to work out for themselves what makes that goal worth achieving'.
>
> Freeth (2002)

NLP can make you an even better leader, whether or not you are in a formal leadership role, by helping you to generate your vision, explore your values and ensure the two are congruent.

Just in case you are not already convinced of the potential value of NLP to you as a healthcare practitioner, there is also a whole range of advantages to you personally from using NLP techniques. We have already mentioned confidence and self-esteem, within CPD, but we cannot over-emphasise the potential value in transforming you through enhancing your belief in yourself. When real change work is undertaken using NLP, people talk of being a 'new person' and of 'starting life over'. We often think it is impossible to change some of those features of personality which appear to be so ingrained that we assume they are just part of us. From personal experience we, as authors of this book, can all give testimony to the fact that even those deep and longstanding aspects of us which we did not like can be lost easily and quickly, with the right person guiding us through the techniques.

Can you see how, by achieving these outcomes, you will be happier and less stressed? And if you recall the strong mind-body link we referred to earlier, you can see how this can make you physically healthier too.

You might read this and think we are either over-stating the potential of NLP or talking about just a few people who experience such radical and life-changing results. It is your choice whether you believe us or not. The only essential ingredient for success is a desire to change, a desire to have more and to achieve more. But don't just take our word for it. Take the opportunity presented in this book and experience those changes for yourself; then share it with others. There may be some people who cannot go through this journey alone and that is fine. We would urge you to find someone to walk the journey with you; find a coach so you don't miss out. This is literally an opportunity to turn your life round; don't let it pass you by.

Making it happen

So, as you are reading on we assume you are excited by the possibilities outlined above and you are willing to take that first step. So how can you make this happen for you? It is essential to remember it can only happen from within. One important concept within NLP is that of 'cause and effect'. Effect is where you blame external things or people for the situation you are in: where work is dreadful because of a bullying boss or because you are not allowed to develop. You are not comfortable in a team because of a particular personality who is unfriendly towards you. Can you perhaps recognise some of these patterns in yourself and your own vocabulary? Are you ever tempted to blame 'them' (whoever they might be) for problems in your life or your workplace? You need to get yourself to be 'at cause'. Cause is where you take responsibility for your own reaction to those external stimuli. You do not condone bullying or harassing behaviour, nor do you allow it to affect you. You try to understand the difficult personality and see the positive intentions of any actions and recognise that the person is doing the best they can with the resources they have. You decide what impact you will allow their behaviour to have on you.

For some people just reading that paragraph will be a huge challenge and if that is the case for you, we suggest that you find a coach to explore the issues it raised in you as you read it.

We believe that by ordinary healthcare practitioners, you and us, taking this seriously and making small changes initially within ourselves, by showing what a difference can be made and enthusing and inspiring others to follow suit, we will transform the environments we work in.

There is a real temptation to think that we are too small, or not powerful enough to make significant changes. Yet it is these very beliefs which hold us back and stop us achieving the changes which will create the future we desire.

We are a small group of healthcare practitioners who have discovered something which can radically change healthcare practice. By reading this book, you become a part of that group. We, both you and us as authors, then are charged with the role of implementing that change in practice. We hope you will come on board and start to make changes at whatever level you are at which will transform healthcare practice both for the practitioners and even more importantly for the patients.

You have already started your journey by reading this far. Keep dreaming your dreams, keep believing in yourself, make the changes you want to make, and watch the positive results unfold around you. You are unique in the set of skills and talents you have. You are powerful beyond your wildest dreams and you can make a difference here and now. Be bold, be strong, and step out to be the expert practitioner you want to be, and enjoy every minute of it.

References

Freeth, P. (2002) *What Kind of Leader are You?* http://www.BookShaker.com, http://www.bookshaker.com/article_info.php?articles_id=118 (accessed 11.05.06).

Knight, S. (2002 2nd Edition) *NLP at Work: The difference that makes a difference.* London, Nicholas Brealey Publishing.

O'Connor, J. (2001) *NLP Workbook: A practical guide to achieving the results you want.* London, Element.

O'Connor, J. and Seymour, J. (1990) *Introducing NLP: Psychological skills for understanding and influencing people.* London, Thorsons.

Self–empowerment

Jim Lister

2

> If you think you cannot succeed the chances are that you will not. If you believe you will succeed, you are already half way there.

This chapter is written for you, regardless of where you are on your own professional development journey, whether you are hugely successful and achieving great things, or whether you are just starting out or feel far from being self-empowered. We want to make you even more self-empowered so that you can be even more effective at what you do.

We make no apologies for focusing on you as a starting point, and throughout the book, and in our conclusion. For so many reasons it is essential to devote time to yourself when exploring professional development. It is only through encouraging, supporting and nurturing yourself that you will become an expert and leader in your field. So yes, this work is about professional development, and its focus is through personal development; it is service development through development of you as an individual.

When was the last time you really sat down and thought about what you wanted from your career? When did you last set time aside to assess where you are on your career pathway and really consider 'what next'? This chapter will help you begin to get to know yourself better, make you more aware of who you are and will help you to take responsibility for the changes which are possible as a result of reading this book. The journey starts here, with you.

A starting point

When I am working with teams of healthcare professionals, I often walk into a room and draw a small dot in the middle of a flip chart pad. I point to the dot and simply say, 'Hi everyone . . . of course it all starts with this, doesn't it?' And people look at me and say, 'What does?' And I say, 'Everything does', and they start to laugh slightly uncomfortably. Then I ask again, 'It all starts here, doesn't it?' Blank looks, and I offer again: 'Everything involved in change starts here . . .' and words start to emerge: 'The NHS, my boss, the universe, us . . . me!' And I say, 'Yes, I think so, and that's where I'd like you to start and end the session . . . with you.'

And as I look around the room I see that most people seem hooked, ready to engage and to contribute. They seem optimistic and relieved that the session might enable them to understand themselves with more depth and insight. It feels like we are on mutually safe territory!

What's so crucial about 'me'?

By emphasising the central importance of me at the beginning of my practical sessions, I invite the participants to begin engaging in the process of self-empowerment in order to further develop their self-awareness. This chapter examines the crucial concept of self-empowerment, and it will inevitably put into place the essential foundations for the remainder of the book, because it explores the core issue influencing how effectively we deal with personal and professional change. And this core issue can of course be expressed very simply: 'me'. This is the 'self', the 'I', the unique entity at the centre of all that is experienced within my existence and being. Self-empowerment essentially involves concentrating during the initial stages of self-development on the role of me being who I wish to be, thereby gradually achieving fuller self-possession, and increasing the understanding and control of our own motives, faculties and capabilities. In looking after ourselves, we become more able to fulfil our professional role as a carer of others.

It is crucial to develop our resources of self-empowerment because so many of our personal and professional problems have their origins in the neglect of 'me'. A quick reflection on some common experiences in the workplace will support this assertion. How many times have you faced change at work, and become derailed from what you want to achieve by the actions of other people? Have you noticed how these people then start to become the focus for our problems? And how we convince ourselves that, if only they would do what clearly they should be doing, everything would be OK? However, we know, when we are thinking rationally, that these people never do what we want them to, but that won't stop us from trying to persuade them and cajole them, and it won't prevent us from fretting about their actions and behaviours and generally allowing them to get under our skin and stress us out!

In other words, although we know that we have to deal with change and its effects, it seems only too easy to fall into the trap of concentrating our energy on a frustrating attempt to change other people. This of course is often fruitless, and becomes the cause of even greater stress. It is more useful to focus our energies on ourselves in order to work through the change, and to become equipped with the tools, the actions, the behaviours and resources that we need to remain effective and to deal with change in a healthy way. Using this approach, we might be able to influence that other person through our own change, through a crucial transformation that we have brought about in ourselves, and through our own practical, visible, demonstrable example of adaptability and efficiency.

To summarise these ideas in the words of Aldous Huxley, 'There's only one corner of the universe you can be certain of improving, and that's your own self.'

Felicity's Story

The experiences of Felicity, a nurse, illustrate the benefits of this process in action. For many years Felicity had carried on with her career, its highs and lows. Suddenly she realised that she needed to take a step back and look after herself: 'For years I was under the misapprehension that my profession would somehow look after me . . . I relied too much on other people, my managers, the politicians. I found myself constantly let down. And then one day the light bulb flicked on in my head – it is up to me! I have to sort myself out to deal with this. And that's where I've been ever since, finding ways to empower myself.'

'Self-empowerment' sounds such a simple concept, and yet it can appear to be incredibly difficult to put into practice. As Felicity found, this is probably down in part to the pressures of modern-day life; humans have never before lived their lives at such a frenetic pace. One obvious symptom of this is that we spend less time just sitting, thinking, reflecting, just spending time with ourselves, allowing ourselves to be bored! We vitally need this 'down time' as it's fashionably called, or my preferred term, as a friend used to refer to it, 'essential, purposeless time'.

What are we up against here?

We have so far established that it will be useful to deal with any change or challenge by starting with 'me'. This approach can be especially useful when we become stuck in a particularly troublesome situation or episode in our lives, stuck in terms of believing we have no more options available to us, stuck in an unhelpful emotional state, stuck in our own low self-belief or fragile self-confidence. It is a rare person who has not at some stage of their lives felt an overwhelming sense of frustration or powerlessness at the sheer complexity of external circumstances, especially perhaps, in areas as complex and sensitive as the caring professions, such as the NHS in the UK, or in any large healthcare environment.

The poet Philip Larkin is especially adept at capturing these moments in modern life, when we feel that our resources and faculties have seemingly become frozen by conditions and events beyond our control or comprehension:

> *Life is an immobile, locked,*
> *Three-handed struggle between*
> *Your wants, the world's for you, and (worse)*
> *The unbeatable slow machine*
> *That brings what you'll get.*
>
> *Philip Larkin*

Now there's a man who can't be accused of being unduly smug! The quotation comes from a poem called 'The Life with a Hole in it', which many of us perhaps at times feel we are suffering from; there is a chasm where our self-possession, our power to shape our own destinies, ought to be.

Whilst we can admire the verbal wit and poetic skill with which Larkin captures this predicament, we would be fully justified in wanting to do everything in our power to avoid being trapped in it ourselves. The techniques of NLP and coaching help us to resist the urge to defeatism or resignation when we are faced by that 'hole' within ourselves and in our professional lives, created by the demands of modern life. So, how do we lift ourselves without having to rely on others to do it, or by waiting indefinitely for more 'favourable' circumstances?

Answering that question is essentially what this book is about. We will now move on to look at practical methods we can use to invigorate our inner resources, bolster our autonomy, and take an independent hold on the circumstances of our lives and our overall destiny. As we have said in the Introduction (Chapter 1), this book will help you to get more of what you want out of life, at home and at work. Engage with it expecting results. Start dreaming of what you will become . . .

Living in cause and living in effect

While it is easy to blame what's around us for how things are, how much more powerful would it be if we took responsibility for those things we could change, regardless of who created them?

Before we embark on the first practical exercise, it is worth just reiterating a useful early principle to bring to your awareness. The concept of cause and effect will help to explain why we often seem hopelessly stuck in awkward problems, and will offer a vital first step in liberating ourselves from these problems. Ever heard yourself blaming others and feeling frustrated because they won't do as you wish? Then read on.

We can spend a great deal of our lives living in 'effect', in other words, dealing with the effects on 'me' and on other people in a situation which hasn't gone the way we might have wished. We choose to do this 'fire-fighting' rather than looking at the cause of the problem. We might ask whether this principle perhaps afflicts the NHS and the wider healthcare profession. Rather than dealing with the core problems of the organisation and the way that it is structured, politicians and managers dream up initiative after initiative to deal with the effects of the core problems. And, perhaps unsurprisingly, the problems are never properly resolved. The core issues remain the same, and we all know the impact this has on the people who work for the organisation.

Far better, then, that we try to avoid this way of living our own lives. Instead, if we can work at 'cause', then we can truly empower ourselves to bring about the adaptations we need to make to embrace the changes that we are involved in. This is a true first step to self-empowerment.

Exercise 2.1
Putting Yourself at Cause

This exercise will increase your ability to see beyond effect, and probe down to the cause at the root of any particular circumstance or problem.

Think of a situation in which you are involved at the moment that feels as if it is having a negative impact on you. Examples might be:

(Children calmy)
(me)

- dealing with a patient who is unresponsive to your ideas
- working with a colleague who is not working as a team member
- a manager who is treating you unfairly

Ask yourself these three questions about the situation:

1. How am I doing?
2. What am I doing? *Getthy cross*
3. Where are things heading? *Gradually improving*

And when you have answered these questions, ask yourself this:

Am I operating 'in effect' (where you will be raising excuses or justifications for your own behaviour)? Or am I operating 'at cause' (where you take responsibility for your actions and you recognise your impact on the situation)?

If you find that you are operating 'in effect', then try and move into 'cause' by asking yourself the following key question:

How have I managed to be part of the cause of this through my own actions, behaviour and decisions?

The information that you will get from this questioning process will start to give you different viewpoints and answers, and as a result will make you feel differently, and will help you to act more positively and constructively.

Consider the example of Helen below, who helped the team that she was advising to overcome some fundamental problems by shifting their focus from cause and move them into effect.

Helen's Story

I was acting as a consultant to a team of ten people whose role was to introduce new working practices in an NHS Trust. Their job was to implement the changes decreed by central Government, working with employees at all levels, from consultants, to doctors, nurses and administrators.

After a few months' work, the group was feeling demoralised. They felt that they had a thankless, almost impossible task, and that they were under fire from all sides. They were encountering objections and opposition from the people with whom they were meant to be working in partnership, and the Chief Executive, to whom the team leader directly reported, never seemed to be content with the targets they had achieved, consistently expressing disappointment at where they had fallen short. Our monthly meetings invariably began with the group offloading their frustrations, detailing the awkwardness and lack of cooperation, amounting at times to face-to-face hostility, that they were meeting as they set about trying to implement the statutory changes.

I realised that the group was dwelling almost exclusively 'in effect'. I was in no doubt that they had justification for many of their grievances; they were a highly skilled team, and they were at times encountering quite petty opposition to their work. Influencing people in the area of change management is never an easy task at the best of times! However, it was clear that dwelling so exclusively 'in effect' was having damaging consequences.

Over the course of two sessions, lasting three hours each, I managed to move the group from being 'in effect' to looking at the problems and challenges 'at cause'. This was brought about in two distinct stages. Firstly, I had the group draw a 'network map', identifying all the groups and individuals they had to communicate with, detailing the links between all the parties. The group specified the types of changes needed for each party, prioritising the significant, influential individuals and departments they needed to get on board. Having assessed what stage they had reached with each of the important parties, the group then had almost a 3D image of what they still needed to achieve, and with whom.

During the second session, I got the group to recognise that it was fruitless to dwell on the things that weren't going to change – external circumstances, the targets, other people. The only thing they could fully influence was their own practice. They had been stuck, caught in a state of overwhelm, but they could now see their way forward. The group spent the rest of the second session devising a well-formed outcome, carefully worded and unanimously agreed. By this stage, they had moved from effect to cause, and they left the session invigorated and with a sense of purpose.

This process helped the group to understand the challenges from the perspective of those who seemed to be creating frustrations and obstacles. They realised that the Chief Executive was being pressurised for results just as they were. The team also recognised that, if they were patient, the employees with whom they were coordinating would embrace the necessary changes with the passage of time as they became more familiar with them and began to understand the benefits and advantages.

The new mindset established in the team brought about significant consequences. No longer anticipating hostility, and armed with an understanding of its causes they stopped encountering it. They began to work in partnership with the employees in the Trust, emphasising the skills that they had to offer in the process of implementing changes. Suddenly, they found that people were now actually requesting to see them, eager to utilise their expertise! This transformation had been brought about solely by the team's ability to move from dwelling 'in effect', to confronting their problems and challenges 'at cause'.

The communication model

We never see reality, for reality is only ever what we want to see.

So, our aim in this chapter is to expand our understanding of how to self-empower, and take responsibility for ourselves in all that we undertake, by operating 'at cause' as often as we are able, rather than 'in effect'. In order to do this, we need

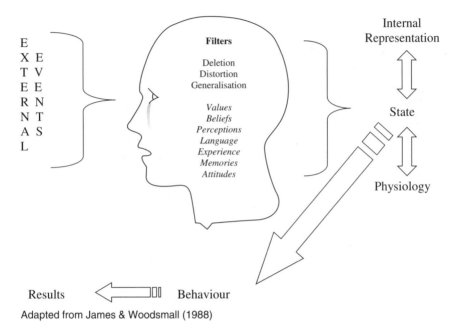

Adapted from James & Woodsmall (1988)

Figure 2.1 The Communication Model

to become aware of how we communicate, firstly with ourselves (truly at cause), and then with others (in effect). Figure 2.1 offers a concise initial introduction to the internal communication process that drives our behaviours and actions.

In summary, this model shows how we process any event through our mind and body, ultimately delivering our external actions, behaviours and results in response to that event. As Figure 2.1 shows we operate a filtering process made up from a number of sources such as our values and beliefs, our memories, experiences, our language and attitudes to life. These filters, unique to each person, then cause us to carry out three functions – deleting (where we literally delete detail from our awareness), distorting (where we misinterpret detail, or make it appear to be something that it is not) and generalising (where we take a small amount of detail and make a broad generalisation about what it means). These three processes are necessary to make sense of any event and to rationalise it, so that we can cope with the sheer volume of information being processed. This mentally edited version of the event, our internal representation (or our map of the world), is given further meaning by blending with, and contributing to, our physiology (our bodies, our physical responses). This combination manifests itself as an overall internal state. This state then drives our actions and behaviours in response to the event, and affects the results we achieve.

Exercise 2.2
Understanding Communication

Now that you have studied the model and begun to understand it in summary form, ask yourself the following intriguing questions:

- How is it that two people can so differently interpret a particular event? For example, any event in the workplace, big or small, a major crisis or a delayed plan, can evoke any number of responses unique to each individual.
- What creates this variance?
- How much control do I have over this process, allowing me to respond and behave in my desired way in any situation that life presents?

Reflecting on these questions should emphasise just how much we all instinctively delete, distort and generalise when we are judging and evaluating our experiences. Remember also that other people inevitably judge us on our actions and behaviours. Yet the Communication Model shows that all our actions and behaviours are motivated through the internal workings of our minds, particularly how we edit, or filter, to make sense of an event for ourselves. We are making judgements only on the superficial information available to us. Hence, it seems very useful to explore how we can become more adept at understanding, and then utilising, this internal representation process, to give ourselves a range of options whenever we act and behave, especially in stressful situations such as those thrown up by work. This will also help us to fully consider other people's actions and behaviours and to think about the deeper values and beliefs which lie beneath.

So we now need to look at the Communication Model in greater depth, in order to find ways in which we can create greater self-empowerment through understanding and controlling both the initial filtering process, and the subsequent elements of our internal representation system.

Deletion, distortion and generalisation

To recap, and to clarify further, the Communication Model shows how any external event, because of the vast depth and variety of the information that it produces, will be interpreted through a series of filters for us to make sense of it. These filters are a mixture of many influences, such as our personal values and beliefs, experiences, memories, language, decision-making processes and culture. These are the things that make us who we are over time. They create our personality and our identity. These filters through which we look at the world, and assess and cope with our experiences, then cause us to carry out three further editing procedures.

- Deletion – where we select some bits of information and ignore others. How often have you been in a crowded room and heard lots of different conversations, and as soon as someone says something relevant to you, like your name, you suddenly 'tune in' to that one conversation and hear it more clearly.

- Generalisation – where we link one or two experiences and draw broader conclusions. An example is where we consider that someone who suffers with Alzheimer's disease cannot give informed consent and then we risk denying those that can give consent the opportunity to do so, by making a broad generalisation about all Alzheimer's patients.

- Distortion – where we make misrepresentations of a reality and form a new 'truth'. This can be useful in a creative sense, for example when we are looking to design a new department and we imagine what it might look like in the future, we distort the present reality, by creating a picture of the new design to test it out before committing to it.

Exercise 2.3
Becoming Aware of our World

This exercise will help you to recognise how you perform all three of these processes quite instinctively, moment-by-moment.

Find yourself five to ten minutes where you can go and sit and just watch an area at work. Find a busy place such a waiting room or a corridor. Notice what you take in through your five senses, what you see and hear, not just superficially, but taking time to notice every detail. Now think about what you can feel, smell and taste, consider each one in turn and really concentrate on the vast amount of information from each sense that is available to you.

Next, observe how your memories and emotions become engaged with this information. Become aware of how much more information you are already taking in about a 'view' which you have probably up until now taken for granted. Maybe compare the image you have now with the image you had of that place before doing this exercise.

Finally, become aware of how you would feel if you experienced everything the world offered with this degree of intensity, not just that one room for five minutes, but everywhere you went, and get a sense of overwhelm!

As you can see, the filtering process is essential in allowing us to make meaning of all that we experience in the world. Without it we would be overwhelmed by the sheer volume and complexities that life presents to us. The 'Becoming Aware of our World' exercise shows how much information is generated even by the most commonplace observations. No wonder our mind says, 'Stop – I can't process all this!'

In order to use this awareness to develop greater self-empowerment, begin to acknowledge how you delete, distort and generalise. It can be as valuable to recognise what we delete, distort and generalise as it is to be aware of the information which is immediately available to us. Start to take notice of this in other people too, especially in their language patterns; for example:

'She hasn't arrived at the meeting on time; she just doesn't care about her job.'

'She is bound to be late, she always is.'

'She has always been like that and always will be. I guarantee it.'

These three statements contain a range of deletions, distortions and generalisations. Are they familiar? Can you identify in each what information has been deleted, distorted or generalised? How useful are they in really understanding and describing the other person? And how many times do we hear ourselves describing ourselves, and one another, in these ways? We can if we choose begin to change the way that we filter and use language, thereby modifying the ways that we respond externally to other people. We can recognise the processes and ask appropriate questions to obtain the information that has been lost or changed. This will bring us a different response and change the results that we are achieving in our lives, for the better. For example:

'She hasn't arrived at the meeting on time – she just doesn't care about her job'

Ask: 'How do you know that her late arrival means she doesn't care about her job?'

'She is bound to be late; she always is'

Ask: 'Always? Can you think of an instance where she has not been late?'

'She has always been like that and always will be. I guarantee it'

Ask: 'How do you know she will always be like that? Can you think of a time in the past when she was not like that?'

By learning to ask appropriate questions, we can break down the filtering process and recognise more easily what has been deleted, distorted or generalised. While it is not always necessary to gain this amount of information, there will be times when obtaining this information could radically change your (or someone else's) internal representation of a difficult situation.

How does the filtering process contribute to our system of internal representation?

To create our total internal representation of a specific event, the filtering process then moves on to the next stage. The edited, filtered representation of events travels internally and is further processed by our physiological make-up, which can vary moment by moment, to create a state (this is how we feel). Whatever state is generated, telling us how we are feeling at any given moment – tired, relaxed, calm, stressed – will then produce our final behaviour. It is that manifestation of our behaviour which determines our results.

Consider a possible example of this process in action. A work colleague has shouted at me. This external event then travels through my filtering process, especially my values, beliefs and past experiences and is internally represented as unfair, and an attack on me. It requires an immediate response. It also happens to be 4.30 pm on a Friday afternoon, and my physiology is tired and de-energised. I have been caught off guard, and therefore my state is one of anxiety, anger and a need to defend. I respond by shouting back, and we have a terrible argument. Could I have responded differently?

Of course I could. Firstly by altering my physiology, perhaps by breathing more deeply, or sitting down. Then, I could have altered the way that I process the event through my filters to allow me to see that this is not a personal attack, simply a piece of feedback which I have to listen to. If I can adapt any part of the internal representation process, it will induce a different state in me, one that for example will allow me to thank them for their feedback, or quietly give them my response. I could alternatively ask them if I could respond on Monday after the weekend when I have had time to think things through. This process of filtering occurs naturally and automatically. By understanding the process we give ourselves the choice of which state we will move into. How useful would it be to you to be able to control your state? What difference would that make to any situations you are currently facing?

Let us now look a little more deeply into how the physiology and state components of the model affect our responses and conduct.

How physiology influences state

Our physiology (our bodily make-up, our physique, our posture, our breathing, our strength, our vision, our skin and bones) is controlled by and controls our mind. It is a two-way process that is inextricably linked. Crucially, we can quickly engineer different and much more helpful, physiological responses to an event by taking action. Here are some strategies that you will find useful:

- **Deep breathing** (whilst meditating). This fills our system with a higher percentage of oxygen, which will change the way we think and will greatly improve our capacity to make quick, clear, rational decisions. This opportunity to step back momentarily gives vital thinking time in order to deal more rationally in today's healthcare environment. By meditating and taking our focus internally, the impact of the external stimulus can be reduced, making it feel more manageable.

- **Regular exercise.** Whether the exercise is walking, stretching or a vigorous game of squash, it will change our physical system for the better. This is particularly worth considering if your role is sedentary and more desk bound.

- **Drink water and eat fruit.** Lay off the caffeine and the fast food for a while, for example one month, and notice the difference in your system, notice how your state alters.

- **Conduct a body scan.** How are you standing or sitting? Change it: sit with your back straight and upright, walk with shoulders and head held high, tilt your chin upwards slightly. Begin to become aware of your posture and change it. Is your breathing aided or restricted by your posture? How might this be useful immediately before presenting yourself at a meeting in order to project the image you wish to project?

- **Change your posture.** If you or your patient get upset, sit up straight, look upwards and smile. Repeatedly (internally) say something positive to yourself. Notice how this makes it virtually impossible to remain in a negative state.

As the model explains, once this physiological response, which we can control to a great extent, blends with our mental internal representation, it contributes to the creation of a state in us. So what exactly does state mean, and are there ways in which we can manage our most efficient state, and therefore control and engineer the most effective conduct from it?

What we mean by the term 'state'

Our state refers to our emotional well-being at any given moment. It is about how we feel. How is it that one morning I can feel strong, confident and ready to deal with anything that comes my way, while the next day all this can have changed and I feel ready to leave my job, downsize my life and run a boarding house somewhere on the west coast of Spain? (Which may be appropriate, if this is a plan driven by my desire to run the best hotel in Spain, but not if it just sounds like a great escape.)

As we have seen, the complex phenomenon of our emotional state is made up of many different elements that all vary at any given time. What I really need to know is how I can actively affect these variables and manage my mood, my outlook and my mindset. Once again we discover that there are many small strategies that, if they are enacted together, can move us from what might be a mildly negative state of mental stagnation and inertia to a far more resourceful and industrious state.

Here are some suggestions for practical exercises that will help you to exert a conscious influence over your state:

- **Stop, sit, close your eyes, and medidate**. Sit and listen, raise your awareness of how you feel, and be aware of your own breathing for five minutes whilst cutting out any other thoughts. When you are relaxed, think how you would like to be: define in as much detail as you can what the state is you would like to have, imagine feeling it this very moment. You will be surprised how you can begin to feel that desired state immediately.

- **Fire some relevant anchors** (see Chapter 8). Anchors allow us to ground ourselves and feel secure in dealing with the issue. They allow us to have our desired state here and now.

- **Play your favourite music loudly, and dance, sing and shout**. See what impact this has on your state.

- **Tell someone you admire them** (one-to-one with care and sincerity). This could be a role model of yours who might then give you ideas about how you could adopt certain qualities of character (or patterns of conduct) to enable you to model the behaviours you value in them.

- **Write down your feelings or draw them**. Use free form rather than going for logical quality – it is the spontaneous act of creativity that matters. It allows us to connect with how we are feeling at that moment.

Bringing together an improved or managed state alongside a greater awareness of our physiology can be a potent tool in self-empowerment. This is neatly demonstrated in an article from the *Guardian* (July 10 2006) written by Craig Mahoney reflecting on the 2006 Wimbledon Men's and Women's Finals:

> 'With players now carefully prepared physically and professionally, the remaining dimension that will distinguish winners from losers . . . is mental and behavioural toughness. The one who on the day is mentally tougher, knowing how to use a range of self-motivation strategies, confidence skills, anxiety control,

and has a sound anger-management structure, will, if they can manage their body, win . . . mental skills will only work if they are aligned to body management, and a convincing posture . . . providing added confidence, awareness and resilience . . .'

Craig Mahoney

The benefits of using the communication model

So what does this exploration of the Communication Model, with all its hidden conscious and subconscious intricacies, mean for our journey towards self-empowerment? How does it help us to choose the kind of behaviour we wish to enact, that leaves us feeling resourceful, healthy and true to ourselves in any given situation? How does it help us to be functioning 'at cause' rather than 'in effect'?

To begin with, the Communication Model raises our self-awareness, which in itself is a useful outcome. This alone will allow us to begin to make some small changes that can add to our self-empowerment. More deeply it allows us to present ourselves with a greater range of options and choices. We can become more effective at noticing our distorting, deleting and generalising, selecting more constructive, liberating filters for our interpretation of events. We can also better understand our values and beliefs (see Chapter 5) and even change them where it is useful to do so.

In addition, by controlling our physiology, we can become more effective at deciding how to influence the subtle internal representations that we make through enhanced state awareness. This will directly affect how we choose to respond through our behaviours and actions, the things on which we are judged. Having greater choices in how we behave, no matter how problematic or threatening, are the challenges that we face in our lives, lies at the core of self-empowerment.

The strategies and tools contained in this book provide the route to becoming who you want to be by achieving the goals that you set for yourself. You will reach this destination through internal and external means: internally by making choices about the way that you communicate with yourself; and then externally, by communicating with others through your behavioural responses.

Here is an illuminating example of someone linking together the components of the Communication Model in order to respond almost instantaneously to a difficult and challenging situation. Consider how you could integrate similar techniques into your own practice, though not necessarily always in such pressurised circumstances as these encountered by Janet!

Janet's Story

I was delivering a paper to 200 delegates at a conference. I was speaking on the perennially controversial subject of change management, and I was fielding questions from the floor at the end of the talk. After two or three straightforward questions, a delegate at the back of the hall stood up, and in a fairly aggressive, confrontational tone, said that he felt that my proposals were totally unrealistic, stating in effect that there was no chance of him putting the projected changes into practice on his own ward.

My response to this challenge was initially the atavistic reflex of defensiveness combined with fear. But I realised almost instantaneously that I did not want to lose my composure and self-possession in front of all these people, up in the spotlight as I was. To do so would undermine the value of my paper, and perhaps set back the progress of the changes I was advocating. I took a few seconds to alter my physiology, breathing deeply, ensuring that both feet were placed firmly on the floor, and facing the audience square on. Maintaining my facial composure, and looking directly at the questioner, I simply said 'Thank you for highlighting the difficulties that still need to be addressed. Your contribution has been very helpful.'

Although these processes were happening over a matter of seconds, and in a pressurised situation, I had reframed the event, applying positive filters to the questioner's motives in making the contribution. I interpreted his comments as being rooted in insecurity about the proposed changes, and as a request for greater reassurance and back-up. These responses bolstered my self-confidence and composure, prompting me to comment to the whole audience, 'This demonstrates that there are challenges still to be faced in implementing these changes,' producing laughter that defused any tension or potential friction from the situation.

My questioner was conciliatory when I met him face to face afterwards, saying that he was simply reacting to the way that I had made the changes sound so straightforward! Not only had a potential conflict of wills been averted, but my use of NLP communication techniques had also reinforced the authority and persuasiveness of my message in the paper about the value of the projected changes to working practice. And in the process I managed to raise a chuckle from my audience!

The culmination of *internal representation*: our *inner dialogue*

To summarise the sequence outlined so far, our filters influence the way that we distort and generalise, shaping our interpretation of events. Our overall internal representation is formed by a blend of our chosen interpretation, our *physiology*, and our *state*. The culmination of this sequence is the language that we use, especially our *inner dialogue*. This language is our self-talk, the internal voice, and it is the way that we judge ourselves, what we say to ourselves about the situations we encounter.

This internal voice is often, strangely, rather harsh. Whenever I comment to people in workshops that we are our own harshest critics, that we give ourselves the hardest time, that we tell ourselves, 'You can't, you are no good, you won't succeed in that,' I see rooms full of people nodding in complete agreement! Wouldn't it be more useful to say, 'I could do that', 'I am capable of feeling the way I want to', 'I can be successful'?

So how can we gain better control of our internal dialogue and language, shaping it to our advantage? A helpful model of internal dialogue is shown in Figure 2.2.

This simple diagram shows how any external response that we make in any given situation is directly affected by the internal language by which we choose to describe it to ourselves, through our actions, language and conduct. Remember this key point, language such as, 'It will be a disaster', 'It's impossible', 'What is the point', 'What a joke', 'I'm not up to this', will probably deliver the result that we are describing – failure by degree. On the other hand, focusing on what is possible, how capable we are, will produce the desired effect as we set ourselves up to achieve our goals.

Bear in mind that we are what we think. Our (external) behaviours, actions and responses are governed by our (internal) dialogue and resources.

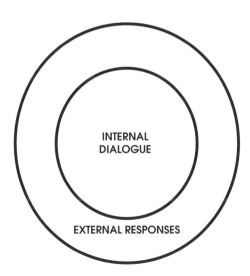

Figure 2.2 Effect of internal dialogue

Exercise 2.4
Hearing Internal Dialogue

This exercise will help you to appreciate the powerful repercussions of our inner dialogue. Take a moment to recall a 'memorable experience', and look again at the previous figure.

Ask yourself the following question: In your 'memorable experience', what resources or qualities of character did you internally request in order to affect your external responses, actions or behaviours? List them under the headings in Figure 2.3.

Internal Dialogue/Language	External Responses
Statements (What you said to yourself, inside)	Actions – what you said, what you did
Questions (What you asked yourself)	Behaviours – how you did what you did
What are your conclusions from this exercise?	

Figure 2.3 Internal dialogue and external responses

Internal dialogue in action

You will begin to notice that your internal dialogue has a number of patterns; that there are statements and questions; and that these statements and questions can be either empowering or disempowering. If they are empowering, our responses will be to go ahead and try out an action. If the statements and questions are disempowering, then they will probably prevent us from taking productive action. They will make us retreat into more defensive responses.

It is clear that our choices of language, essentially our statements and questions, are highly influential in deciding our internal representation of any given circumstances. Clearly, if we learn how to shape and manage the patterns of our internal dialogue, we can significantly increase our control and influence over challenging situations (Figure 2.4). A hypothetical example of internal dialogue in practice will illustrate this key point.

Imagine that your manager has presented you with a new structure for your ward. You must now take responsibility for the plan and begin to put it into place.

Disempowering Internal Dialogue	Empowering
Typical Questions	
Why us?	How can I make this work?
Why me?	
Why doesn't the management consult us?	
Why do they think this will make any difference?	
What is the point?	How can I become involved?
Typical Statements	
This is a disaster	This might make a difference
This won't make any difference	
I haven't been involved properly	
Typical – too little too late	Some of this could work
We've tried this before	
I can't really be bothered	
I've got enough to deal with	I can make time for this

Figure 2.4 Disempowering and empowering internal dialogue

As you can see, the more conscious we become of how we use internal language to describe our potential responses, the more control we will have over its influence. If I think that the change will be pointless and will not succeed, especially as I wasn't consulted ('Why wasn't I?'), the more likely it is that it will become a self-fulfilling prophecy and will not succeed. I will thereby have contributed to my own self-disempowerment. If I can learn to find and then use language, especially internal dialogue, to find different ways of describing how I feel about a situation, ways which will allow me to see possibilities, to have a go, to think it might work, then the more likely it is that circumstances will work out in that positive way that I desire. I will have self-empowered 'me' for a healthier, more productive outcome.

Sarah brought about a fundamental improvement in her life as a result of reviewing and altering the workings of her internal dialogue. Once you have read her account, consider ways in which you might adopt similar approaches when faced with the kinds of challenges you encounter:

Sarah's Story

I had been employed by the NHS for many years, working predominantly as a lecturer, tutoring and mentoring healthcare professionals, advising employees at all levels on how to shape their careers and how best to direct their skills and resources. It was a post that I felt suited me, for which I had been trained, and at which I felt I had achieved a degree of success.

My department then underwent a prolonged two-year review, towards the end of which I began to feel deeply, and for me, uncharacteristically, demoralised. I felt that my role at work was being eroded, and it became clear that, even if our jobs were to be retained, our roles would be significantly changed. The sense that the work I had been doing for many years was now deemed worthless undermined my confidence on every level, spinning off into other aspects of my life – my role as a wife and mother, my self-confidence in all areas.

My internal dialogue became exclusively negative. My head became full of statements like 'You're not worth anything', and every idea seemed to start with phrases like 'You'll never be able to . . .' The questions in my head were full of panic – how could I find a new job at my age, how would I be able to keep supporting my family . . . ? I knew that I was starting to act like a different person, and I seemed to have lost my sense of logic, my self-belief. The lack of communication, the isolation from colleagues caused by the review, seemed so unfair to me and to the unit, and I felt I had no options left, overwhelmed by circumstances.

Then one day, while listening to a life coach addressing one of my groups, I had a 'light bulb moment'. The coach asked the group a direct question, 'What will you be doing in three years' time?' Instinctively, I said to the person next to me, 'I won't be doing this.' Something inside me had prompted me to take possession of my own future, rather than waiting for events to take their inevitable course.

I knew what qualities of character I had to look for internally – determination, logic and practicality – and the nature of my internal dialogue changed. My inner statements now emphasised the skills and accomplishments I had built up during my years of work, and my questions were concerned with how I could now utilise these abilities, and adapt them to the evolving work environment. These statements and questions in turn led to direct action. Looking again at my CV I realised I had worked for and achieved everything there. Even during the course of the review I had completed a Masters degree in Education, and had published a book. I recognised that I had built up a range of unique skills, and that it was now up to me to find the best way in which to utilise them.

By making a conscious effort to shape and control my internal dialogue, my entire outlook was altered. My sense of self-worth, and even self-preservation, was restored, and I felt free to concentrate on the jobs I was happiest doing within the confines of my role. Employees were still eager for my advice, and when I began to put out feelers for alternative work, I found that people were interested in what I had to offer. As often happens when you have a confident sense of purpose, fate intervened for the better, leading me into a new freelance career in which I am using to the full, and am indeed still adding to, the skills and knowledge accumulated during the previous years of my working life.

The sting in the tail

You will only be able to begin to make this adjustment to your internal dialogue if you commit to change, desire it and keep working at it. You need to believe in yourself and your own ability. If this is an issue for you we would urge you to see a coach who is qualified in change work who can help you to take on new, more empowering beliefs and let go of older, less empowering ones. It is like working at any physical change, we exercise hard in the gym to improve our body strength. We need to show equivalent reserves of mental discipline if we are to create empowering internal dialogue, thereby achieving the improvements in attitude and performance that form our key goals.

If I can begin to ask myself empowering questions more often than not, backed up by empowering or affirmative statements, then I will begin to find answers. It is worth noting that the answers that are generated by empowering questions might cause us some discomfort by moving us out of our familiar or habitual patterns of thinking.

An example might be, if you were to ask the following disempowering question:

'Why does my manager always pick on me?'

This can be moved into an empowering question:

'How can I work more effectively with my manager?'

The answers that might be generated could include:

Ask for more regular one-to-one meetings.
Give my manager more up-to-date feedback about progress.
Present my case in a different way.
Take my manager for lunch once a month!

Exactly how palatable these options might be will inevitably depend upon your criteria. Perhaps the lunch might be a bridge too far, at least in the first month of your new relationship!

This example begins to show us that true self-empowerment can and should lead to new actions. These actions will reinforce our commitment to the changes we have set in place, ensuring that we maintain momentum. However, it does not preclude the likelihood that these decisions and actions will be complicated and will provide us with challenges. We are not pretending that self-empowerment is always easy; but it can be! You are already beginning to focus on what it is you wish to achieve, who you want to be, and striving for the goals that you have set yourself. Start to develop a positive internal dialogue you can repeat frequently to yourselves to take you forward towards your goals.

Exercise 2.5
Working at Cause

This exercise will bring together in practice all of the ideas covered in this chapter.

Step 1
Think of a work-related issue that is causing you some degree of uncertainty. It might involve other people, individually or in teams. It might be recent or longer term.

Now notice how you feel, and write down key words or phrases.

Step 2
Work now with cause and effect. Ask yourself these questions:

'What is it about me that is making me feel this way about this situation?'

'What have I done to help create this situation I am now involved with?'

Listen for your responses and if it helps, write them down.

Notice how you feel compared to when you began this exercise. Do you notice a difference?

Step 3
Look at the situation and discover how you have formed your opinion or your standpoint. Ask yourself these questions:

'What have I missed here through my generalising, distorting and deleting?'

'Can I begin to use this new information to change the way I see things and to change the way I feel?'

Listen to your responses and if it helps, write things down.

Step 4

Listen to your internal dialogue. Write down typical self-talk, both questions and statements. Distinguish between what you would consider to be empowering and disempowering language.

Start to move the disempowering questions and statements into more empowering questions and statements.

Once you have written them down, read them out.

Notice how this feels. Are you able to convince yourself to take any new action that is suggested by the empowering answers that you are now providing yourself with? Are these possible solutions palatable and realistic?

After taking these four steps, sit back and reflect on how you feel. Are you able to further boost yourself with a quick state and physiological change? Take some exercise, play some music, enjoy an energising drink or simply sit up straight and look upwards and imagine how good things could be.

Should you feel sufficiently changed to begin to move yourself forward into action, then begin the change. After some time, notice how long this change lasts and how energised you remain. How long is it before you need to further boost yourself?

Repeat as required.

Summary: the centrality of self-empowerment

This chapter has provided a detailed definition of self-empowerment, emphasising that starting with the self is an undeniable first step towards coping with challenges and the demands of change. We have seen how acknowledging the central priority of taking care of 'me' is a vital initial step towards gaining greater self-awareness, and understanding ourselves as expert practitioners and leaders. This idea will be critical when we move on to Chapter 6 on Perceptual Positioning where we see the significance of the first step, to decide what my own needs are and to determine my best intentions in any given situation.

We have also looked at the principle of seeking to live our lives 'at cause' rather than 'in effect' wherever we are able. It is more empowering for me to find out how I might have been part of the causes of any given situation, no matter how negative. If I can become clear about this I can truly adapt and change for the future. If not, the problems will probably produce recurring patterns and I will spend my life dealing with the effects and consequences. Even now can you recognise recurring patterns in your life that you would wish to avoid in the future? Moving from effect to cause might take some time, but the more we practise the principle, the more effective we become and you might find that you are pleasantly surprised at how easily you can make that transition using the tools outlined in this book. We encourage you to start to take responsibility for yourself, to start to get the results you want to get.

We have become familiar with the Communication Model that all human beings use to make sense of the world, and which in turn makes us the unique individuals that we are. We have shown how this broad, common communication process inevitably dictates that we will experience any event differently from other people, no matter how close we are to them; family, friends, work colleagues within and outside our profession, whoever. This model has shown us that if we become aware of our filters, how we delete, distort and generalise, then if we choose to, we can begin to use these reflex processes to our advantage, rather than allowing them to control us.

We also explored the two inter-related concepts of 'state' and 'physiological awareness'. If we can use simple strategies to change and control the way we feel both emotionally and physically, we will become more confident and energised, increasing our commitment to the process of self-empowerment. We have also recognised that this set of techniques will produce quick and productive changes, but that these will inevitably take us out of our comfort zone. Working with these strategies will inevitably require commitment and dedication if we are to achieve the kind of enduring, fundamental impact we wish for in our lives. Make sure you put the support you require in place to make the changes you want to make.

Crucially, the Communication Model has also shown us how significant is our 'internal dialogue and language' in the way we communicate to ourselves and create internal messages that shape our actions and conduct. This often harsh voice, our self-talk, is a key indicator and controller of how we deal with difficult situations. Through an awareness of the way language works for us and inside us, either in an empowering or a disempowering way through the statements and questions that we choose to use, we can exert a significant influence on how we operate in the world.

It is difficult to overstate the importance of this process of exerting control over the language that we use to ourselves. As Mary Daly wrote, 'The liberation of language is rooted in the liberation of ourselves.' Although this observation originates from 1973 in relation to the Women's Liberation movement, it is equally applicable to any circumstances in which people are striving to take back power and control over their own lives and destiny. It is equally applicable to you as you look at your role in healthcare, both now and in the future.

Here are a few last reflections that might provide a little final impetus to your desire and determination to engage in the process of self-empowerment. There are many smaller-scale, immediate reasons why we would want to empower ourselves, such as to solve a demoralising work problem, to go for (and get) the promotion we desire, to achieve a more satisfying work/life balance, to gain more control over relationships or domestic circumstances. It can be a tremendous relief and satisfaction to overcome these short-term challenges, using self-empowerment to work towards our broader career and life goals. However, when I am faced with an awkward, difficult and persistent challenge, I bolster my determination to face it not only by imagining what it might be like to be free of this problem, but also by taking a broader perspective, in fact, a much, much broader perspective! I remind myself of, or read again, the following invigorating lines from Bill Bryson's Introduction to his superb 'rough guide' to science, *A Short History of Nearly Everything*:

> 'Not only have you been lucky enough to be attached since time immemorial to a favoured evolutionary line, but you have also been extremely – make that miraculously – fortunate in your personal ancestry. Consider the fact that for 3.8 billion years, a period of time older than the Earth's mountains and rivers and oceans, every one of your forebears on both sides has been attractive enough to find a mate, healthy enough to reproduce, and sufficiently blessed by fate and circumstances to live long enough to do so. Not one of your pertinent ancestors was squashed, devoured, drowned, starved, stuck fast, untimely wounded or otherwise deflected from its life's quest of delivering a tiny charge of genetic material to the right partner at the right moment to perpetuate the only possible sequence of hereditary combinations that could result – eventually, astoundingly, and all too briefly – in you'.

Looked at from this perspective, does it not seem intolerable to even contemplate allowing a single moment of our existence, what Philip Larkin calls 'the million-petalled flower/of being here', to be spent trapped in petty disputes, in various states of resigned frustration, or in mental and emotional inertia, when in reality we possess the power and inner resources to free ourselves at any time? You are the only one who can control your destiny. We hope the fact you are reading this book means that you have already made the decision that you want to be even more successful. Working out how to empower yourself is the first crucial step to achieving that, and you are now ready to take that newly empowered you and create the future you desire. Have fun!

Before you start to read the next chapter just take a moment to write out a list of at least three empowering statements to say to yourself every morning. Once you have done this, commit them to memory, place them somewhere that you cannot miss them each morning, let them become your reality. Over time add new ones. Start to change your internal dialogue here and now, it really is as simple as that to take the first step. What is it you want to hear about yourself that would empower you? What would help you face your day? Maybe pick from the statements below, or create your own, which will really give you what you want.

> I can cope with anything work puts before me today.
>
> I am great at my job.
>
> I have all the resources I need inside me to deal with everything I might face.
>
> I can make a difference.
>
> I am gorgeous.
>
> I am a valuable member of the team.

Create the future you want, become the person you want to be. It starts here by telling yourself what you do want to be.

References

Bryson, B. (2003) *A Short History of Very Nearly Everything.* London, Black Swan Books.

James T and Woodsmall W (1988) *Time Line Therapy.* Capitola, California Meta Publications.

Larkin, P. (1988) ed. Thwaite, A. *Philip Larkin: Collected Poems.* London, Picador Books.

Empowering yourself to others

3

Suzanne Henwood

The greatest discovery you could make is that by making changes within yourself you can change the world

In Chapter 2 we showed you the NLP Communication Model and emphasised the need for self-empowerment, and you will have already begun to think about what you want your future to look like. We looked at the importance of your physiology and how this links with your state, how you feel and your internal representation of reality. This process is important because it is the combination of these three components which determines our behaviours, our outcomes and therefore our results.

In this chapter we want to focus again on you, on your physical self-awareness, your body language, your eye movements and your use of language, and how you build rapport with others. We want to develop what you learned in Chapter 2 and spend some time looking in more detail at how you can change specific aspects of yourself to alter your behaviour and improve your results, and in doing so see how you then change the way that others perceive you. To at least some degree, all of us are concerned with how we come across to others. This chapter will help you to portray the image you want to portray, to give the level of service you want to give. People will create an internal representation of you anyway; how much more effective would it be if you helped to generate that internal representation to ensure its accuracy, if you allowed patients and colleagues to see your care and compassion and your attention to detail? This is your chance to think about how you want others to perceive you.

Rapport

Establishing rapport is probably the single most important skill that you can learn in order to gain trust and respect from patients, colleagues and friends. You will know yourself just how important it is to be able to get alongside, for example, your patients, and in many cases establish very quickly a level of trust which allows them to divulge to you very personal and often intimate details which they may never have shared with anyone else before. How valuable would it be to you to be able to make that connection, very quickly, with each patient that you see or treat? And how much easier and more effective would your job be if you had that skill?

So what is rapport?

Ellerton on his website (www.renewal.ca) says that rapport is the basis of any meaningful interaction between two or more people. He goes on to say, 'For me, rapport is about establishing an environment of trust, understanding, respect and safety, which gives a person the freedom to fully express their ideas and concerns and to know that they will be respected by the other persons'. In healthcare to be able to do this between practitioner and patient or between two practitioners is essential.

The Department of Health on their website (http://www.dh.gov.uk/PolicyAndGuidance) state that the two major complaints from patients concern communication and customer care. Patients want to feel they have been listened to and their concerns and fears heard. By learning and using the skills outlined here concerning how to build rapport, you can ensure that you should never have a complaint filed against you for poor communication. You can also ensure that you give the best possible level of service to the patients you care for.

When you are in rapport with someone, a patient, colleague, boss or friend, you step into their shoes for a short time and you understand what it is they are hearing, feeling and seeing. You may not agree with what you perceive there, but you understand it from their perspective, and this one small step will drastically change the way you communicate with them.

How do you know if you are in rapport?

When you are in rapport with someone you both feel comfortable. You are able to contribute freely to the conversation and you feel at ease, you can relate to the other person and you feel a connection with them. You will find over time that you will 'match' their body language and gestures. We all do this unconsciously in our everyday lives, though we may not be aware of it, and we can harness this deliberately in order to speed up the process of building rapport to ensure a great outcome for our patients and for ourselves.

How do you establish rapport with someone?

In order to establish rapport you need to get into the same state of mind as the other person. Pay real attention to things like how they are sitting or standing, how they are holding their heads and their body positions, the words they are using and how they are using their voice and in some small way try to replicate that, without obviously mimicking them. This will help to put you into a state of rapport with the other person.

If you have a frightened patient in a wheelchair, who has been brought to you for a consultation or treatment, you cannot possibly even begin to know how they are feeling until you get into their 'state'. Sit alongside when you talk to them, so you are on the same physical level. Consider what it is like not being able to get up and walk away and how that would make you feel; consider what it is they are in hospital for and what feelings might go alongside that possible diagnosis. If the patient has been brought from a ward, consider the uncertainty they might be facing in being brought to a new department, possibly with little warning or explanation of what to expect. Consider also how you might feel walking into, or being wheeled into, your department for the first time. Perhaps take a few minutes one day to walk in, or be wheeled in, from the main door, and really notice all that you see and hear. If you were not familiar with the environment and the people within it, what might make you nervous or uncomfortable? What would make you feel at ease?

Another aspect to consider is to match the energy level of the person you are establishing rapport with. If someone is really angry and/or agitated, you will not establish rapport by trying to talk to them slowly and softly. Match the energy level, without aggression and without any threatening wording, then gradually once you have the rapport, you can slow things down and 'lead' them to a calmer state.

Note of caution

If someone is in a negative state, you clearly don't want to match that exactly, so match some elements purely so you can then lead them out of it. Meeting anger with anger will not be effective. See Richard's Story for an example of where this was successfully used by a radiographer who learnt the technique of establishing rapport.

Richard's Story

Richard is a radiographer. He frequently works in the accident and emergency department and recounted an incident where he was met with some aggression by a patient who felt she had been waiting too long for an x-ray.

Richard was working alone, and returned to the department, having been in theatre. On arrival at the department he was met by a patient who asked in an aggressive manner, 'Where the hell have you been?'

Richard had been on duty for eight hours prior to going on-call. He was then five hours into his on-call shift and he had not had a proper meal break.

He realised that giving the patient excuses or trying to explain where he had been would not be effective until he had established rapport with the patient and got the patient into a better state.

The patient was talking quite fast, in a higher than normal tone and appeared agitated and was moving around as she spoke.

Richard immediately apologised for keeping her waiting, making sure he matched the tone and speed of her voice. As he unlocked the department he asked some basic questions about what she was waiting for and said how he would now focus all his attention on to her.

As she realised he was taking her seriously, she calmed down a little as she was led to a more positive state by Richard talking just slightly more slowly and calmly.

By the time Richard has processed her request form at the computer, throughout which time he continued to talk to her, and led her into the examination room, the patient was calm and apologetic for having been so 'mouthy' when he first arrived.

Richard recognised the components of the patient's state and the way this was being demonstrated in her vocal speed and tone. He matched the speed and tone, being careful to use gentle, positive language and then gradually led her to speak more slowly and calmly. He established rapport and gained her trust.

If Richard had responded with, 'I was in theatre . . . I have been at work for 13 hours without a break', all true and all good reasons why he was not present when she arrived, why he was cross too, the chances are he would not have calmed the patient down, he would have escalated her frustration and probably matched her negative state. As the professional practitioner, he recognised that it was his responsibility to manage her state and not to reveal the negative components of his own; he was working 'at cause' (See Chapter 2).

Exercise 3.1
Building Rapport

Find a colleague who will get involved in an exercise with you. Explain to them the outline of rapport and explain that the exercise is designed to try to show how using rapport changes how you feel in any situation.

Agree a mildly controversial topic to discuss.

Start to talk about it and agree with what your colleague is saying about it. While talking deliberately try to mismatch your colleague so that you are not in rapport. If they are standing still, move around; if they are talking in a high tone, talk in a low tone for your normal range; if they are sitting with their legs crossed and leaning back, uncross your legs and lean forward.

Let the conversation continue for a few minutes.

At a convenient point change your point of view so that you now disagree with the other person but start to build rapport.

Let the conversation continue for a few minutes.

Finally, have a few moments of both agreeing and building rapport.

Stop the conversation.

Talk about how each 'section' of the conversation felt.

Take a few moments to reflect on how this might be useful to remember in your own areas of practice. Think about times when you might be out of rapport with your patient due to what you are doing, for example positioning someone in imaging or preparing a sterile trolley, and consider what you could do to establish rapport in sometimes less than ideal circumstances, for example talking with someone lying on a bed.

Learning how to establish rapport could be one of the most beneficial skills you can develop to make your patient's experience even more positive. As well as providing a comfortable environment emotionally for your patient you will also increase the chances of obtaining the information you require to treat the patient effectively, so we would urge you to increase your own awareness of when you are in and out of rapport and how you can change that to get the results you want even quicker.

Physical self-awareness and body language

You may be wondering why the inclusion of a section on body language is essential in a book about self-development. Are you aware that only about 7% of your communication depends on the actual words you speak? A study conducted in the 1970s by Mehrabian (published in 1981) which has been frequently repeated and verified and showed that the vast majority of your communication is non-verbal, and a large part of that is your body language, alongside tone of voice. So when you greet a patient for the first time, what does your body language communicate to them? When you talk to them what does your tone of voice convey? Are you clear that what is conveyed is the same as what you would wish to be conveyed?

Here we will look just at body language. There are many components of body language that we could discuss, but here we just want to alert you to some very common ones. By being aware of these components of body language, and using them effectively, you can really help to present yourself more effectively and significantly increase the chances of getting the desired outcome.

One word of caution: body language can be misread. You can put your own map of the world on to others and we have to be cautious about generalizing too much in listing common considerations. What is important is to get to know the person, know what a particular movement means to them and look for other clues to confirm your assumptions. Let me give you one personal example. I often sit with my arms folded, even when sat comfortably at home watching TV. I also fold my arms when I am thinking something through, especially when I am thinking what to say. I worked for a short time with a management consultant who was adamant that my crossed arms meant I 'had got to my limit', to use her words. She interpreted what my crossed arms meant in her map of the world, without taking into account my normal behaviour, my other signs, or indeed my ongoing positive involvement in meetings. Initially I laughed and pointed out that while we make generalisations about some particular gestures, we must be careful not to over-generalise. She genuinely misread my gesture on numerous occasions and actually antagonised me several times by insisting she was right when I had actually been in a good state. While we would advocate that you take time to be more familiar with common gestures and what they might mean, we would urge you to use this in conjunction with other clues and use feedback from the other person to assess whether or not your reading of the situation is actually correct.

In the light of that note of caution then, here are a handful of common gestures which might indicate particular meanings or states:

Eye contact

In the UK we expect to have eye contact with others. Be cautious, as this is not always the case in other cultures.

For those who expect good eye contact, it shows interest in them and respect. It can even be interpreted as a guide as to whether or not someone is trustworthy. In a health environment it is important to establish and retain good eye contact with someone to whom you are, for example, imparting important information, or with someone from whom you are trying to gain trust. Consider the possible negative effects of:

- recording in a patient's notes while you are speaking or listening to them;
- watching a VDU while talking or listening to patients;
- positioning a patient or setting up equipment whilst introducing yourself or giving information or advice.

It would be worth considering how both your clinical activity and maintaining good eye contact can be achieved simultaneously, or the absence of eye contact explained so that it is not misinterpreted.

Position of your head

The position of the head is an easy gesture to use in healthcare. If you want to be respected and seen to be an authority on something, try maintaining a level head position, so your head is pointed straight towards the person you are with, and neither tilted chin up nor chin down. If on the other hand you wish to make a closer contact with a patient, you want to show you are listening, try tilting your head slightly to left or right, and move it occasionally to the opposite side.

Position of your body

The angle of your torso can be an indication of your feelings and attitudes towards another person. If you tilt your body towards someone you are likely to be interested in them, or in what they are saying. If you are very short on time and need to finish a consultation at a point when you have obtained all the information you require from the patient and the patient has got all the information they require, then by tilting back slightly you will introduce a distance and break your intense interest in what they are saying, which will indicate that the consultation or conversation is about to end. You can use this personally for time management too, when you wish to resume work once someone has come along to ask you something.

One of the best reasons to understand and be aware of body language is to help you establish rapport quickly and easily with someone else. In NLP this is termed 'matching and mirroring'. Taking care not to openly mimic the person you are communicating with, just as with voice speed and tonality which we discussed earlier, observe a particular aspect of body language and subtly mimic it in some way. This can be done by matching or copying a movement. Have you ever noticed when you are in the bar after work with colleagues, how if one person goes to lift a glass to drink, others will also raise a glass shortly afterwards? You can spot leaders of groups in this way and watch who it is who is influencing the group. Alternatively you can mirror movements to be even more subtle; this is where you copy with a similar movement, but maybe with a different body part, for example, mirror a foot tapping with a hand movement, as opposed to matching like with like. If a patient is agitated when speaking to you and is tapping their foot or bouncing their foot up and down, just gently tap your finger on the table, or tap it on your other hand, at the same speed, until you feel you have rapport, then 'lead' them by slowing the pace. If you are in rapport, their pace will also slow and as that physical gesture changes, so it will impact on their internal state and consequently also their behaviour – think again of the Communication Model. You are then more likely to get the results you require from your interaction. You will be surprised just how effectively this establishes a deep connection with another person.

It is worth saying that you will find with body language that 'a little goes a long way'. Use subtle, small gestures and do it with the intention of helping the other person, not to manipulate or mimic them. Watch and listen. You will be surprised how much you learn about your patients and colleagues, from practising and becoming proficient at using these techniques.

Eye accessing cues

Another useful component of body language for us to use in our communication is the position of the eyes when talking and processing information. The position and movement of our eyes can give huge insight into the way we are thinking. Whether we are relating to what is happening around us or whether we are focusing on our own internal feelings and images; the position of the eyes shows whether a person is thinking visually, through sounds, by self talk, or through how they feel. This is done automatically and subconsciously and most people are unaware that their eyes are even moving in relation to their thinking patterns.

If you wish to build rapport with someone, one of the most effective ways of doing so would be to 'match' their thinking style. By watching closely for eye movements, which are often subtle and quite rapid, you can add to your tool box of communication. This will enable you to establish a real connection with another person and ensure you get the best possible information from them, by using this information to decide on the most appropriate language to introduce. For example, if you can see from their eye movements that a person is visualising and using visual processes, it would be far more effective when speaking to them to say something along the lines of, 'I see what you mean', than to say, 'I hear what you say'. This is particularly important when you want to let a patient know you are listening to them, that you have heard them and that you do understand what they are trying to express. If you use the wrong language they will not feel like they have been heard, regardless of what you said, or how you felt the interaction went.

Eye positions

So what are we looking for? There are predominantly six main positions outlined in Figure 3.1 below (originally mapped in NLP by Bandler and Grinder, though discussed by various authors from as early as the 1890s). One important point to note is that for a small percentage of people (approximately 10% and linked to a large extent to left and right handedness) the positions are reversed. This is not too important in establishing whether someone is visualising or using auditory language and processing. As you will see below there are two of each of those positions. In the case of self talk and feelings though, you might need to see how someone responds to your initial guess as to which language is appropriate, and change it if necessary. In some contexts, where you are likely to spend more time with a patient, some simple questions would establish this for you to ensure you are correct. For example asking them what colour their car is would establish visual recall as opposed to visual construct. The question 'what would your car look like if it was covered in pink spots' would give visual construct.

Why is this knowledge useful to have in your tool box?

In the context of healthcare, why is it important to have this tool available? Below are some ideas of where you might use this information in practice:

- It will enable you to build rapport with others more easily, quickly and effectively by matching their thinking patterns.
- You can also use this knowledge to help you and your patients get the answers you are looking for. For example look up and left if you wish to recall something that you saw, and you will find you recall it more easily. This is a great tip for students if you are helping them in clinical practice to recall something they may have seen before or learnt in class. To recall something you heard, look left and sideways, which is great to help a patient if they are struggling to recall something they have been told. Another example of this is to encourage someone who is upset to stop looking down where they are accessing their feelings. By moving their eyes upwards you will reduce the intensity of any negative emotion and increase their ability to tackle the situation in hand.
- If having explained something to someone and they say they do not understand and are looking up, they are trying to visualise the outcome. It would be worth offering to demonstrate for them as they may need to see you do

something before they can process what you are saying. This also is great for working with students.

- In giving feedback and responding to people, try to match their patterns. To praise a visual person try, 'That looks great', whereas to someone with an auditory preference you might say, 'That sounds great,' and to a feeling thinker, 'That feels great'. This can be a really effective way to relate to and motivate your staff and students in the right context.

- Be confident enough to allow people time to think and respond. If you see that the person to whom you have asked a question is moving their eyes around, they are thinking through their response. By interrupting them to request a quick response, you will interrupt their thinking. Give them the space and time they need.

- Give information in an appropriate way. If you can see the preferred way of thinking of a colleague or a patient, by reformatting any information to fit their preferred style, they are more likely to take the information on board. For example, for someone who is visual, ask them to picture something or ask if it is clear. For someone who is using an auditory style, ask them if they have heard what you said. For someone highly kinaesthetic, ask them how they feel about what you have told them. They will want to be involved, and they will also appreciate having something they can physically take away and hold, maybe an information leaflet for example. For those who display evidence of self talking, give facts and evidence to support what it is you are telling them and ask them to think about what you have told them.

- Consider how this might relate to the issue of personal space. For someone who is highly visual, they will want to see you and take in information, so you would be wise to sit further back when talking to them, whereas someone who is predominantly thinking in feelings will want to be close enough to be able to touch you.

- To establish how someone makes decisions or learns something new. By talking through a process of, say, learning, get someone to recall something they learned effectively. You can establish the stages of learning for that person so they can deliberately retrace those steps when faced with something new to assimilate. This enables even more effective learning in the future.

- Influencing. People tend to have an eye spot for particular responses, for example saying yes and saying no. They also tend to have an eye spot for people they like and dislike. Establish where their eye spot is for their favourite person, perhaps by asking them questions about their favourite footballer or actor, then having established where they look when talking favourably about that person you know where to stand, in that line of sight, to influence how they perceive you too. Similarly, if you want someone to agree with you make sure you stand in their 'yes' spot; again watch their eye movements when they are in agreement and when they are not in agreement.

All of these uses take practice. You cannot expect immediately to be able to use the full range, or notice every indication. We suggest you pick one and practise looking for it and then try a different one the next day. You will find in time that it becomes more natural and almost second nature to build this information into the wealth of data you take in about any interaction.

Just a note: if you are struggling to build rapport with someone, or you find being in their company uncomfortable, it is worth considering whether you are using opposing thinking preferences. Be aware of your own preferences, as well as the preferences of the people with whom you are communicating. If you find that you are in this situation, try to alter your use of words to match their preferred thinking pattern and you will be amazed at just how quickly you can build rapport and start to communicate more effectively. Be flexible. Again, as the professional, take responsibility for matching those thinking patterns to establish rapport; don't expect others to match you.

So what are the eye movements?

The movements are described here from the other person's perspective, so remember this is their left and right, not your left and right as the observer (Figure 3.1).

Remember also that if the eyes are looking straight ahead, but not focusing on anything in particular, or they appear to be dilated, the person could be accessing any of the six sensory areas, although it is more likely to be visual than any other single area being tapped.

Also be aware that regardless of the question you ask, the person could reinterpret that question internally and use their preferred patterns of processing that information, before replying to you. For example, if you ask someone who is strongly visual what is their favourite pop song, they may initially visualise the artist, so their eyes may initially go to visual recall. If you are not sure, just ask them what went through their mind in response to the question.

As you look at the other person:

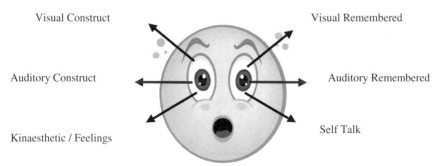

Visual Construct   Visual Remembered

Auditory Construct   Auditory Remembered

Kinaesthetic / Feelings   Self Talk

Figure 3.1   Eye movements

Two very nice websites which allow you to interact with models and see for yourself how eye movements occur can be found at: http://www.mindworks.uk.com/website/eyecues.htm and http://www.nlpweekly.com/files/NLP_Weekly_Eye_Accessing_Cues.swf

---

Exercise 3.2
Working with Eye Patterns

Find yourself a partner and sit opposite them. Ask them the following series of questions and for each one observe their eye movements. See which direction their eyes move in, remembering that some people's eye movements will be more obvious than others, some will be faster than others, so you may have to ask a couple of questions to convince yourself the movement was not just a fluke. Once you are convinced of the direction of movement, move on to the next set of questions – you do not need to ask all of the four questions for each position. You will find a blank response sheet on the website at www.wiley.com/go/nlphealthcare

1. **To assess Visual Remembered:**
    1. What colour is your front door?
    2. What colour is your favourite mug?
    3. What colour uniforms do nurses wear?
    4. What was the last thing you watched on TV?

2. **To assess Visual Construction:**
    1. What would your uniform look like if it was bright pink?
    2. What would your staff room look like if it was painted with green spots?
    3. What would your best friend look like in a red wig?
    4. What would the waiting room look like if it was full of comfy modern sofas?

3. **To assess Auditory Remembered:**
    1. What does an emergency bleep sound like?
    2. What sort of ring does your department telephone make?
    3. Can you think of someone with a very distinctive laugh. What do they sound like?
    4. Has a patient or colleague ever shouted at you? What did they sound like?

4. **To assess Auditory Constructed:**
    1. Can you imagine the sound of people in the waiting room singing?

   2. What do the sound of a heart monitor and a dripping tap sound like together?

   3. What would your receptionist sound like if she spoke like Mickey Mouse?

   4. Can you imagine what you would sound like if you had a very high or low voice?

5. **To asses Auditory Digital (Internal Self Talk):**

   1. Just listen to your own internal voice for two minutes. How do you know it is your voice?

   2. When do you talk to yourself?

   3. What do you often say to yourself, inside?

   4. Just say to yourself, 'I am good at my job'.

6a. **To assess Kinaesthetic Remembered:**

   1. What does it feel like to hold a newborn baby?

   2. What does it feel like when someone you help really expresses their gratitude to you?

   3. Can you remember the last time you felt really good about some aspect of your work? When you knew you had done a really good job?

   4. What does it feel like to be called out in the middle of the night?

6b. **To assess Kinaesthetic Construction:**

   1. Imagine the feeling of cotton wool turning into a glass beaker.

   2. Imagine the feeling of skin turning into water.

   3. What would it feel like if when you were really angry about something you turned that anger into laughter and joy?

   4. What would it feel like to feel really tired, after a long shift, then suddenly feeling full of energy and really motivated to do something exciting?

Points to remember

* A small percentage of the population will be reverse organised.

* A small percentage of the population will have linkages between the positions, so that to access visual language they have to feel something first for example, so if eyes dart around consider a linkage between systems.

* If a person has a very high tendency towards one particular way of thinking, they may go immediately to that system regardless of the question asked. If you are unsure, ask the person what went on in their minds in response to the question.

Judith's Story

Judith is nurse in cancer and palliative care. She is a trained counsellor and uses her counselling skills in clinics to help patients, particularly those who have just received a positive cancer diagnosis.

Judith was in a clinic with a patient, Mary, who had just been told she had breast cancer. After the consultation, during which Mary had seemed to cope very well, Judith asked if she would like to talk through the treatment options which had been explained to her. Mary, along with her husband, moved to an adjacent room and sat informally to talk. Mary appeared to try to put on a brave face and told Judith all was well, she would have the recommended treatment and she would get through. Judith felt that she was acting as if she was trying to give her husband support, he had gone very quiet; she did not feel Mary was truly expressing herself.

Judith, reading Mary's non-verbal communication, recognised that she was distressed, and while talking to her recognised that she was accessing the visual eye areas. She started asking her questions like: 'Do you see any problems with what is being proposed?' 'What support would you like to see in place to help you through this?' By talking Mary's visual language, Judith broke through the barrier of self-protection, and Mary started talking more openly with her. Although she went through a period of time very distressed as she faced up to her true feelings, she left the department having got the support she required; she left knowing she had been listened to.

Start to practise using eye cues, take more notice of eye movements in your interactions and enjoy the increased flexibility it leads to as you adapt your style to create even better rapport and even more effective communication with patients and colleagues.

Linguistics

Understanding the power of language and how it makes us feel could literally transform us and those we come into contact with.

This last section is a brief overview of some of the language patterns which can be so incredibly powerful at changing states and interpretations of reality. In Chapter 6 we will look at the technique of 'reframing', whereby changing the way something is described can change how things are perceived.

Here we are going to look at some specific language patterns which can be used easily and effortlessly, which could transform potentially difficult situations and change how you feel and how you are perceived by others. It is not possible here to fully explore the power of language, and we would urge you to read around this subject more fully. What we hope to do here is raise your awareness of the possibilities of the power of language, to open up your map of the territory just a little. This will help you start to listen to yourself even more effectively, both internally and externally, and to start considering how the words you use transform the meaning of any communication which occurs.

Let me introduce a huge word to you, a word which can open up minds and can make all sorts of things possible which seemed impossible. Just one word. Can you think what it might be? 'No', your internal dialogue may have responded here. How does that make you feel? Like giving up? It probably does not make you feel like looking for where the answer will be. What about if when I said, 'Can you think what the word might be?' instead of your internal dialogue saying, 'No', it says, 'No, not yet'. How does that change your feelings about whether or not it is worth trying something else to think of the word or it is worth digging deeper within yourself for the answer. Just using the word yet can change the perception of whether or not something is possible. Whether or not it might happen but has just not happened **yet**.

Let's look at some potential scenarios we might face daily

Within teaching:
Lecturer: Do you understand?
Student A: No (left with potentially feeling 'I am hopeless or stupid').
Student B: No, not yet (leaves the way open for understanding to come, could even lead on to the student saying, could you just go over that again? I haven't quite got it yet). The expectation is that they will understand in the future).
Lecturer: You got 40%, you have not passed yet. This implies there will be another opportunity to re-sit an exam and that the expectation is that you will pass it next time. Clearly this is more empowering to the student, although we do recognise that there are a limited number of attempts allowed in which to pass an examination in most clinical courses.

Within clinical practice:
Patient: Has the chemotherapy worked?
Doctor A: No, unfortunately not (leaving patient deflated and full of concern).
Doctor B: Not yet (leaves the patient with some hope and a view that something else will be tried. Clearly you would not want to give this impression if you had genuinely come to the end of the line in options available).

Just take a few minutes to think about where you might in the past have used the word no, when adding 'yet' to the end of the sentence could give the person you are communicating with, including when you are inwardly talking to yourself, more options and the opportunity to keep trying.

Can you begin to see the care with which we should choose our language? So, let's just look at two more words which can easily be used interchangeably and which give a very different feel to any conversation.

Let's look at a patient complaint. A very distressed patient approaches you, clearly agitated, and verbally throws a complaint at you. Think of what sort of complaint could be forthcoming in your own department. Just imagine what it feels like to be that patient, get up and walk through how you would be feeling, what you would be preparing to say, how you would say it. You are angry, you feel let down, maybe you are frightened. Now read the following responses from staff and see how you feel after each one:

- I am sorry, but I am not the right person to talk to.
- I am sorry and although I am not the right person to talk to, I will get my manager for you.
- I am sorry, but I am with another patient right now.
- I am sorry, and I am with another patient right now, can you wait for a few minutes?

By changing one word can you feel the difference? Can you recognise what the word 'but' does in the sentence? It completely negates all that has gone before it. Your mind concentrates only on what comes after the word 'but', whereas with 'and' you acknowledge and retain what was said in both halves of the sentence.

You could of course add other softening words, for example:

- I am sorry, I can see you need to sort this out and I am not the right person to talk to, let me go and get my manager so she can resolve this for you right now.
- I am sorry and I am with another patient right now, could you bear with me and just wait a few minutes so I can make sure she is safe? I will come right back to you.

Just take a few moments and consider where this might be useful:

- When you disagree with someone you could acknowledge what they say and then suggest an alternative.
- When you don't feel someone has done enough, you can agree with them and then suggest additional action on top of theirs, not instead of.

Of course you can also use 'but' effectively, when you want to disregard what has gone before.

- 'I can't offer you an appointment on that day, but I am going to do everything I can to get you an appointment at a convenient time.'
- 'Yes, the NHS is experiencing a lot of difficulties at present, but we have implemented many new policies to start to turn things round.'

Think about what message you want to give and ensure you use the most appropriate words.

Here are some other brief examples of how changing one word can change how someone perceives what it is you are saying:

- Can you come to my office, I really need to talk *to you* about something?

  Compared to:

  Can you come to my office, I really need to talk *with you* about something?

By changing the word 'to' to 'with' you take away the potential feeling of threat, the feeling that you are going to be chastised about something when you go to the office.

- I am sorry *my* staff did not provide the service you required today.

  Compared to:

  I am sorry *the* staff did not provide the service you required today.

By introducing the word 'my' in this context, the manager takes ownership and becomes part of the staff group. When using the word 'the' she distances herself from the staff. She may also imply a lack of emotional involvement in the issue.

And finally, think about the effect the word 'try' has on your internal representation:

Clinician: I really need that new piece of equipment in place by Friday.

Equipment rep: 'I will try.'

How much faith do you have that the equipment will be in place? Very little. If you apply this to yourself, and also remember the NLP presupposition which states that you get what you focus on, then if you are asked to do something you might avoid using the word 'try' as the chances are you will still be 'trying' at the deadline. As a manager you might watch out for this and recognise that someone who says they will try to do something for you is maybe not either fully committed or they do not believe in their own ability, so need extra support or time. By overcoming this at the time of setting up any agreement, you set yourself up for success.

While we cannot cover all aspects of language here, we wanted to raise your awareness around issues of the power of language and how we might utilise it to our advantage in our practice. As Rudyard Kipling said, '*Words are, of course, the most powerful drug used by mankind*'.

Before we close, we also just want to raise the issue of the use of language and its effect on health, disease and healing. Again this is a huge subject and we want to do no more here than raise your awareness and spark your interest in this area. Just spend a moment thinking about some of the language you hear from yourself, from colleagues and from patients.

- I need a break.
- This really eats away at me.
- I have had a gut full of this.
- He broke my heart.

'Organ Language' such as this can indicate that there is a mind-body link occurring, which the patient may not even be aware of. There is also a real chance that if you say these things to yourself, your mind will work to act them out in practice. You may find that you return from holiday with a broken bone if you went for a break. Someone who presents with stomach problems, such as ulcers, may have felt that something was eating away at them. Can you think what associations may occur with the other two statements, and also any other statements you remember hearing in your own practice?

Another area closely associated with this is the language and phrases used within clinical practice, which might set up a negative response in patients:

- My/your bones are crumbling.
- The cancer is eating away at me.
- It may leave you with a nasty scar.
- You could be in for a rough few months.

Can you think of alternative ways for either expressing these sentiments, if they are said internally, or for you expressing them differently if they are words you would use yourself in practice?

- The bone structure has been affected and we can work to reduce the impact of that and ensure it does not continue.
- The cancer has affected some other cells and we can prevent that from continuing by . . .

- We will do what we can to make the scar as small and unobtrusive as possible.

- It may not be an easy time and we will do all we can to support you at every step.

By carefully thinking about the words you have used and the construction of the phrasing, you can prevent what is known as 'installing' a response into the patient. If a patient believes their bones are crumbling, what impact will that have on their life? If they are aware there is a structural issue which is being treated, how differently would they respond?

Now that you understand the structure of internal representations and that language is one of the filters to those representations, it is worth taking some time to listen to the words being said, so that you can choose the words you use even more carefully in the future.

It is clear that NLP gives us the ability to understand the power of language and the impact that language has on our behaviour and results. Start to listen out for language which may not be positive, which may be exacerbating a condition or which is not giving the patient the positive resources they require to achieve healing. Listen to the words being said and reflect on how those words might be interpreted. You could change the way you talk to patients and you could change the way patients talk to themselves in order to increase the chances of positive results.

One final word on language and the way something is said. If you have negative internal self talk which you would like to eradicate, think about changing what you say and the way you say it. Try saying the following phrases sounding like Mickey Mouse or Donald Duck:

You don't really know what you are doing.

Nobody likes you.

You will never achieve anything.

Try standing up and saying them again while looking up towards the ceiling and smiling, maybe even add 'oh no no no no' at the end of the sentence. You may find just by using your knowledge of the Communication Model and applying that to your use of language you can change your internal representation of yourself as a result. How good would it feel to be able to disregard those negative internal voices which disempower you? Conversely, start to build up positive messages to replace the previous negative ones. Say the positive ones with sincerity and start to change your beliefs about yourself, from the inside out.

By reading this chapter you are already thinking about the power of language and how you can make changes in your own use of language to empower yourself and to change the way you are perceived by others. You will be surprised just how effectively people pick up on your new internal dialogue and start to perceive you differently, once you look at yourself in a new light. Use what you have learned here to put across to colleagues and patients the projection of you that you want them to see. Make sure you leave others with your desired impression of who you are and what you value.

In summary

This chapter has looked at a variety of ways to increase our self-awareness and how we can change the way we are perceived by others. We have raised a number of issues, which we hope will spark your curiosity. You are probably already considering when you can find out more about these issues. We would urge you to start playing with, and practise, some of the concepts we have introduced here. Start to watch actions and listen to what is being said, both internally and externally, in a new way. Start to raise your awareness of your reactions to what you see and what you hear and reflect on how things could have been done or said differently to get a different result. Enjoy your new heightened awareness and use it to make a positive difference for you, your colleagues and your patients. Start to make small differences that will really make a difference in your practice.

References

Department of Health (http://www.dh.gov.uk/PolicyAndGuidance/OrganisationPolicy/ComplaintsPolicy/NHSComplaintsProcedure/NHSComplaintsProcedureArticle/fs/en?CONTENT_ID=4081003&chk=8sU8KJ (accessed 23.09.06)

Ellerton R *Rapport*. www.renewal.ca (accessed 23.09.06)

Mehrabian, A. (1981) *Silent Messages: Implicit communication of emotions and attitudes.* Belmont CA, Wadsworth.

Taking control of your life

4

Liz Holland

Taking the first step is what is really important. By taking the first step you realise the variety of paths ahead from which you could choose.

Introduction

This chapter is to enable you to put into action some of the thoughts which are now going round your head about things you would like to change. How many times have you returned home refreshed from a holiday feeling determined to change something in your life? How many times have you heard about a new technique and not applied it to your practice in the long term? How do you measure your own level of motivation towards making any changes and how useful would it be to have a set of tools which enables you to really take control of you life. This chapter will give you those tools.

When we are aware that we want to make some changes in our lives, whether at work or in our private lives, it is easy to proceed with great enthusiasm and then for our progress to gradually slow down as day-to-day activities take over our lives, or we run across obstacles which seem insurmountable, or we just run out of steam. This is similar to having good intentions when making New Year resolutions. We resolve to do something or cease to do something on January 1 and by February 1 our good intentions have not been acted on and we have continued our usual patterns of behaviour.

Many people wait until there is a critical incident in their lives before they make the changes they had been considering, but had not put into action.

A major change in health, death of a loved one, divorce, redundancy, promotion, having a baby and forced changes in the workplace are all examples of critical incidents that tend to force people to re-evaluate how they are living their lives. But why wait until you have a critical incident before living the life you really want?

Health and safety in the workplace are important issues world-wide. Employers are now required to provide and maintain a safe work environment for their employees. Health and Safety in Employment Acts in the UK, USA, Canada, Australia and New Zealand include stress as one of the factors that employers must take into consideration when developing their policies and procedures. Work stress and stress-related conditions are the second most commonly reported work-related illnesses in the UK. An estimated 12.8 million work days are lost every year to work-related stress, anxiety or depression (HSE, 2004). Reported stress is found to be highest in teachers, nurses and managers (Smith *et al.*, 2000). UK physicians are reportedly at particular risk of experiencing depression; and increased use of alcohol is a commonly perceived solution used to cope with events in their professional and personal lives. Some of the preventative measures suggested to combat stress at work include career counselling, coaching, counselling and psychotherapy (Firth-Cozens, 2003).

This chapter is written to assist you in taking control of your life now, this very moment, not waiting until you have a critical incident that forces you to make changes in a less than ideal environment. The exercises can be used for your own reflection or as a discussion point with your coach or clinical supervisor.

We have found the following tools effective for assessing our current state, how we feel, and finding what part or parts of our lives need our attention. While there are other tools available, we share these as ones which have worked well for us and our clients.

The four tools presented in this chapter are:

- The six-step change process: to give you an overall process to follow for any change you want to make
- The Wheel of Life: to assist you in gathering information about your life
- 'Begin with the end in mind' visualisation tool: to assist you in knowing what you want in life and what 'success' means for you
- The 'CCCSS Model': an additional tool to assist you in evaluating what is important in your life right now

Use these exercises as a starting point, so you can begin living the life you really want to live.

Where to start: the six-step change process

1. Gather information about your current situation.
2. Select the areas that you want to make changes in.
3. Consider a number of possibilities that could be options for you.
4. Develop a plan through establishing goals (refer to Chapter 7).
5. Action your plan.
6. Monitor your progress and make adjustments as required.

The Wheel of Life

Exercise 4.1
The Wheel of Life: Gathering information about yourself

A very useful tool to assist with evaluating satisfaction levels in your life is called 'The Wheel of Life' (Whitworth *et al.*, 1998). The 'wheel' is divided into different areas to represent different aspects of life (see Figure 4.1).
   Suggested labels for the wheel include:

   I. Career – your current occupation
   II. Personal Development – developing your capabilities to reach your potential
   III. Physical Environment – the place you live
   IV. Friends and Family – you may wish to separate these into two different areas on your wheel
   V. Romance/Life Partner
   VI. Finances – your income, expenditure, savings plans
   VII. Fun and Recreation – how you spend your leisure time
   VIII. Health and Fitness – your physical/mental/spiritual/emotional well-being

The wheel is used by placing an 'x' on each spoke to signify the degree of satisfaction you are experiencing with that aspect of your life. If the x is near the centre of the wheel, then there is little satisfaction, and if it is on the outer edge of the wheel a high degree of satisfaction is being experienced. If it is helpful you can score each area out of ten, where zero would be at the

centre of the circle and ten would be on the circumference. The score represents a subjective measure of your satisfaction and in order to calculate it
you might like to consider issues around your actual performance and your
own expectations of performance in each area.

Once an x has been placed on each segment, join the lines up and
imagine that wheel rolling along beneath you. Would you get a smooth
ride?

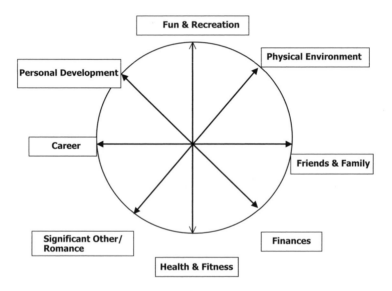

Adapted from 'Wheel of Life' (Whitworth *et al.*, 1998)

Figure 4.1   Wheel of Life

You will also find a blank Wheel of Life on the website at www.wiley.com/
go/nlphealthcare. You can use this as it stands or you can adapt the labels to
areas which are more relevant to your own life.

Anne's Story

Anne is a 45-year-old Registered Nurse. She filled in the Wheel of Life, and it looked like this:

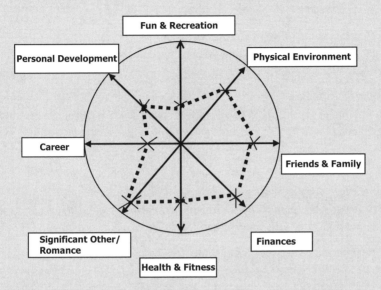

Figure 4.2 Anne's Wheel of Life

Anne followed the six-step change process:

1. Gather information.
Anne completed the Wheel of Life.
   When Anne discussed her Wheel of Life she said her current workload was overwhelming. She acknowledged that her job gave her the opportunity to have a pleasant home, and she was reasonably satisfied with her income. However the shift work and extra workload she carried meant that it impacted negatively on her health and fitness as she had no energy left for exercise at the end of her shift. On further questioning, Anne disclosed that she had been diagnosed with diabetes within the last nine months and also had elevated blood pressure.

2. Select the areas that you want to make changes in
Until Anne had completed this simple exercise, she had not realised that she had been focusing on earning extra income to reduce her mortgage rather than acknowledging the need to take care of her health.

3. Consider a number of possibilities that could be options
Anne brainstormed all the possible options she could consider to look after her health and still maintain her preferred lifestyle. She then identified which options she was prepared to take immediate action on, and others that she will put into place in a manageable timeframe.

4. Develop a plan through establishing goals
Anne developed a plan of action to assist her to achieve her goals. (Refer to Chapter 7 for one method of setting goals.)

5. Action your plan
Anne commenced her plan immediately. The plan included regular monitoring of her health with her GP, and Anne recorded her sugar level, weight and blood pressure in a diary to record her progress towards her longer-term health goal.

6. Monitor your progress
Anne reviewed her plan once a month with her coach. She found that her original plan was over-optimistic, so she made adjustments that were more realistic.

Result: Anne developed a plan of action to take care of herself, and her coach assisted her in keeping on track. Anne was a person who benefited from having to show her diary record to someone else on a regular basis to avoid slipping back into her former habits.

Adapting the Wheel of Life for more information

The wheel can be used as a starting point to assist you in knowing what you want in life and what success means for you. It can be used in many different ways. As well as an overview of different areas of life, the labels can be changed to look at the different roles you have in your work (see Maureen's story later in this chapter), and different roles you have in your life, such as partner, parent, friend, team, group or club member.

You can then either:

- assess the satisfaction you are gaining in each of these roles or
- assess the approximate percentage of time you are spending in these different roles.

Let's look at some examples.

Mark's Story

Mark developed the following list of life roles that were important to him:

- *Partner*
- *Father*
- *Son*
- *Uncle*
- *Nephew*
- *Health professional*
- *Chairman of a School Board*
- *Student – completing postgraduate studies*

These roles were used as the labels on his Wheel of Life and his assessment was the degree of satisfaction he was gaining from these different roles. His self-assessment showed that he gained satisfaction from his work, study and his School Board but little from his personal relationships. One of the conclusions he reached was that he did not put the time and effort into those relationships as he did into other activities. He developed strategies to enhance his personal relationships, as that was the area where he wanted to make significant improvements. To do this, he used the 'Begin with the end in mind' visualisation tool (See Mark's Continuing Story on p. 74).

Maureen, whose story appears below, used the Wheel of Life to assess her different work roles. It was a starting point that enabled her to evaluate her work, and to assess whether she was using her time effectively.

Maureen's Story

Maureen is the manager of a Radiology Department. She identified her ten main work roles as:

1. *Staff recruiting, contract negotiating and orientation.*
2. *Establishing and monitoring budgets.*
3. *Managing quality systems.*
4. *Facilitating staff meetings.*
5. *Representing Radiology at other hospital-related meetings.*
6. *Developing staff rosters.*
7. *Controlling stock control and related invoicing.*

8. *Writing reports and submissions.*

9. *Executive member of her professional body.*

10. *Member of a group monitoring training programmes.*

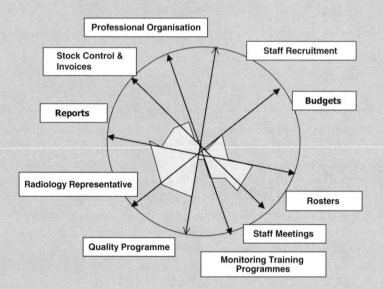

Figure 4.3 Maureen's Wheel of Responsibilities showing percentage of time spent in different work areas

Maureen followed the six-step change process.

1. Gather information:

Maureen kept a time log for over a month to assist in more accurately estimating how much time she was spending in each activity. To do this, she developed a single sheet of paper with the ten areas listed down the side. Each evening before leaving work she recorded her estimate of the time she had spent on those activities that day. At the end of the month she tallied up the times.

She noted that she didn't have to monitor a training programme during that specific time period, and made allowances for this in her final calculations. She then had a 'best guess' at how she spent her time on this activity in other months when training was running.

2. Select the areas that you want to make changes in

Maureen reviewed her different activities and considered that some were essential for her role as a manager, but others could be performed by other people.

3. Consider a number of possibilities that could be options

Maureen asked herself the following questions to assist in clarifying possible options:

- What activities do I like/dislike?
- What activities will I be expected to do whether I like them or not?
- What risks do I have to consider if someone else performs these activities?
- If I make any changes, what will be the best use of my skills and experience?
- What delegated activities will assist towards covering me when I take annual leave?
- What skills and experience do other staff need to acquire to assist with succession planning?

4. Develop a plan through establishing goals

Maureen identified potential staff that she thought she could delegate new responsibilities to. After gaining their acceptance, she developed a training programme for each staff member and estimated the time it would take for her to deliver the training and monitor it. (Refer to Chapter 7 for a suggested way of establishing goals.)

5. Action your plan

Maureen put her plan into action.

6. Monitor your progress

Maureen found that a new project she was involved in impacted on her time available to actually teach the staff their new responsibilities. She realised that if she did not make the training a high priority, she could still be doing tasks in six months' time that did not require her attention.

Result:

When Maureen assessed the percentage of time she spent on different roles, she quickly identified the areas that demanded a large proportion of her time. Through this simple analysis, Maureen identified the roles that were important for her to continue to take responsibility for, and those for which she needed to train other staff to manage. Maureen trained one of her clinical staff to take responsibility for the rosters and one of her administration staff for the stock control and invoicing. She also reviewed the meetings she attended and dis-cussed with the person she reported to which were of value and which meetings she no longer needed to attend. Having a visual tool to show her manager assisted the conversation they had.

Maureen gained 24 hours per month to spend on higher priority roles and her administration staff enjoyed the extra responsibilities they were given.

Begin with the end in mind

In his book *The 7 Habits of Highly Effective People* (1989) Stephen Covey includes a chapter entitled 'Begin with the End in Mind'. Here he provides a visualisation exercise that encourages people to imagine attending their own funeral and listening to speakers from four different groups (family, friends, colleagues, and church/community organisation) talk about them. The exercise is to identify what you would like these speakers to say about you and your life, to highlight what is important to you. In imagining what you would like them to say, you can start developing a personal frame of reference. Developing this framework can assist you in making decisions and making a positive impact on your daily behaviour so that it can 'fit' with what people may say about you and your life at your funeral. This concept of 'beginning with the end in mind' can then be useful in clarifying your values and what success means to you.

Exercise 4.2

How to apply the concept of 'beginning with the end in mind' to your daily life and using your 'Wheel of Life'

Step 1: Identifying the different areas in your life

- Look at the labels on the sample 'Wheel of Life' on p. 66.
- Do the names of the labels suit your situation and cover all aspects of your life? If not, change the name on the labels to make the wheel more meaningful for you. For example, you may want separate labels for 'family' and 'friends' or add 'community service'.

Step 2: Focus on one area of your life

- Select one of the areas of your life from the wheel to think about.
- Find a place that helps you relax, whether it is sitting by a fireside, being out fishing or running, lying in the sun on a beach or sitting in your favourite chair.
- Turn your thoughts to this area of your life, and imagine that you have achieved all your dreams and goals in this area. You have been very successful in this area of your life, and you feel very proud/content with your achievements. What would your life look like? What would you be saying to yourself? How would you feel? Allow your thoughts to flow freely.

Step 3: Record your ideas

* Once you have thought about this area of your life, take out a large piece of paper. In the centre of the paper write the name of the area of your life that you are evaluating.

* Draw lines outwards like spokes from that word and record the thoughts you have had of how you really want this aspect of your life to be. Write as much detail as you need to describe your thoughts, feelings and desires.

* At some point turn to Chapter 5, and read about values. Will your professional and personal values be met in the ideas you have recorded? Use your values to give more depth to your ideas. It would be worth returning to revisit this record when you have identified your work values as it may impact on the results here.

Step 4: Visualise living your life the way you want it to be

* We describe a number of visualisation techniques in this book, for example, Mental Rehearsal (Chapters 8 and 9). Read these to either refresh or teach yourself the technique.

* Picture yourself acting, thinking and feeling successful by your own criteria in this area of your life.

Step 5: Act as if . . .

* Start acting as you have visualised yourself to be. Are your actions showing you being your 'best' self? Would someone observing your behaviour be able to correctly assess what values are important to you?

* Use the visualisation you have created as a reference point. For example, if you are making a decision, ask yourself whether it will fit with your visualisation of who you want to be.

Focus on your next area

Now that you have developed the technique, select another area of your life from your 'wheel' and follow the same process.

Developing each area of your Wheel of Life takes time. It requires you to clarify your values and what you need to feel successful and satisfied in different areas of your life. Use the values elicitation tool in Chapter 5 (Exercise 5.2) for each area of life you explore.

Mark now continues his story to illustrate how he applied this technique to improve his relationship with his partner.

Mark's Continuing Story

Mark identified from his Wheel of Life exercise that he was not satisfied with some of his personal relationships. He acknowledged and took responsibility for the fact that he spent less time and energy on these relationships than his professional activities. Mark started thinking about what he wanted from his life partner. He wondered what it would be like if he had a partnership that was really great instead of one that he admitted he took for granted.

Having a coach provided Mark with time and a confidential environment in which he could talk about his ideas. I asked him what he needed to feel loved. What did his partner need to feel loved? Mark had no idea, so I gave him 'The 5 Love Languages' by Gary Chapman (1995) to read. Chapman identified that people can express their love for someone in five different ways. As the person experiencing the feeling of being loved, we may have a preference as to what is important to us. Chapman called the five 'languages':

1. *Words of affirmation*
2. *Receiving gifts*
3. *Quality time*
4. *Acts of service*
5. *Physical touch*

Mark assessed himself as a person who gives gifts as his main expression of demonstrating his love for someone. He talked to his partner about the book and discovered that she felt loved when Mark spent quality time with her. Mark realised that was the one thing he was not doing. This conversation with his partner was a turning point for Mark. It got him thinking about what he needed to feel loved, and what he wanted from his relationship. He allowed time for reflection and did not rush this process. He observed other people's relationships more closely, and also started talking to his partner about what they wanted. As a couple they started communicating at a different level, and each used the 'begin with the end in mind' technique to clarify their thoughts, expectations and dreams. As they became clearer about what they wanted, they would discuss their findings. Mark was amazed at how his attitude changed towards his life partner through these discussions. He found this exercise enlightening and a vehicle for talking about issues that he would normally struggle to talk about. As he found out more about himself and his partner he acted differently and therefore took a step closer to making his visualisation a reality.

Mark's story illustrates other essential points that are worth exploring if we want to make changes in our life. Firstly, we need to be aware what needs are not being met. Mark's awareness was created through his Wheel of Life assessment and talking to his partner about both his and his partner's needs. Secondly, we have to know what it is we want so that we can develop a plan to make the desired changes. The final step is that we need to act on our plan to make the change. These steps can be summarised in the formula:

Awareness + Self-knowledge + Intention + Action = Change

The CCCSS Model

Another starting point for gathering information about yourself is a very simple assessment of your present situation. Ask yourself a question, and then apply the CCCSS Model to find your answer. An example is given in the next exercise.

Exercise 4.3
The CCCSS Model

Question: If I looked at my present situation, what do I want to:

C – **Continue doing**, because it contributes to my having a fulfilling life and contributes to my life's purpose?

C – **Change**, because I could improve these aspects of my life?

C – **Complete**, so I gain a sense of accomplishment and have more time and energy for other things in my life?

S – **Start**, because these things will contribute positively to my life?

S – **Stop**, because these things are no longer contributing to my life or stopping me being the person I want to be?

An example of how this can be used is illustrated in Paul's story.

Paul's Story

Paul is an Anaesthetic Technician who was recently promoted to a supervisory role, which he is finding challenging. He lives with his partner, and his partner's two children. Paul was feeling somewhat overwhelmed when he decided to find a coach. He was asked to think about his daily activities and interactions with people, and then analyse these activities following the CCCSS Model. Paul was given the CCCSS worksheet and asked to identify at least two to three activities in each category.

This is what he brought back to his next coaching appointment:

Identified Activities

C	**Continue**	○ Attending professional development courses
		○ Regular work out at the gym
		○ Having an annual holiday overseas
C	**Change**	○ Formal communication with staff needs a different strategy
		○ How I react to stressful situations
C	**Complete**	○ Final paper to achieve my postgraduate qualification
		○ Renovation of kitchen and laundry
S	**Start**	○ Performance reviews with staff
		○ Involving others in key decisions at work
		○ Improving relationship with partner's children
S	**Stop**	○ Smoking
		○ Watching so much TV
		○ Taking so much work home each night

The worksheet proved a useful starting point for Paul. He identified what were high priority items for him; what action he could take immediately; what activities he needed to develop strategies to achieve the results he wanted. Paul used his coach for this process, and his coach helped him keep on track. Some of the items on the list were a real challenge for Paul, so being able to talk with a confidant and develop achievable goals assisted him greatly. (Refer also to Chapter 7 for goal setting and Chapter 9 for managing stress.)

Taking control of your life right now

> Those who get on are those who tend to get up and get on with things, creating the future they desire.

We want you to be the person you want to be, and live the life you really want, at home and in work. We want you to have increased self-awareness, feel motivated and to be happy. Not tomorrow, but starting right now!

How often have you heard people say, 'I'll be happy when. . . .'

- I've paid the mortgage
- I've obtained my goal weight
- I have a partner
- I go on holiday
- I have the job of my dreams
- I have my own apartment/house
- I've travelled around the world
- I have . . .

Psychologists are turning their attention to the science of happiness, and researching what makes people feel fulfilled and happy. Dr Martin Seligman has worked for more than 40 years on the science of optimism, learned helplessness and depression. He is now considered the 'father of positive psychology' and his books and website (http://www.reflectivehappiness.com) give practical exercises to assist in building happiness. The benefits of happiness are said to include greater productivity and higher quality work, more satisfying and longer relationships, more friends, stronger social support, bolstered immune system, lowered stress levels and less pain (Lyubomirsky, 2005).

These are attractive benefits, so what attention are you paying to your happiness?

Here are eight practical suggestions, adapted from Sonya Lyubomirsky, for taking responsibility for your personal level of happiness:

1. **Count your blessings**. Look for the things that are going well and acknowledge them in your life. Record the things you are grateful for in a journal. They may be very simple things such as being able to enjoy a tea break with your colleagues, to more significant events of recovering well after surgery. Every day say thank you for three good things which have happened that day.

2. **Pay attention to the small joys in life.** The sound of birdsong in the early morning when you have been called into work; the drawing your three year

old gives you; the feeling of the sun on your back as you walk to your car after your duty has finished; a genuine smile or 'thank you' given by a patient. See '10 Delicious Daily Habits' p. 179. This exercise assists you in appreciating small things on a daily basis.

3. **Practise acts of kindness**. Random acts of kindness are encouraged, such as spending an additional five minutes hearing about your patient's great-granddaughter that they had seen for the first time that week; or more regular acts, such as having an elderly relative over for a meal each week; feeding the neighbour's cat when they go away or writing a letter of condolence when someone you know has had someone significant in their life die, or giving a word of encouragement to a colleague at work.

4. **Thank someone who has been your mentor or done something significant in your life.** Don't wait until that person dies before you talk about the positive impact they have had on you. Ring, visit or write a letter to that person now, and tell them how their support has been significant to you and just what a difference they have made.

5. **Take care of your body.** Eating well, exercising regularly, getting plenty of sleep. Take some of the advice that you hear yourself giving your patients! Be a role model for them. Again, '10 Delicious Daily or Weekly Habits' can support you in achieving this. See p. 179.

6. **Develop strong relationships with friends and family.** With modern communication you can still develop and maintain relationships with family and friends even though you do not live near each other. Learn how to text, blog or podcast so you can 'talk' with the younger members of your family; email or telephone those friends and family you cannot see regularly. Learn how to talk with, and listen to, your life partner.

7. **Develop strategies for the tougher times in life.** Pay less attention to your thoughts and more attention on your actions and behaviours. Chapter 9 includes guidance on how to develop a stress management plan. We and our clients have also found it useful to read what we have recorded in our journals in the 'count your blessings' exercise during a tough period in our lives. It reminds us of some of the simple things that bring joy, and they can inspire you to look for small blessings to support you during the challenging phase you are experiencing.

8. **Learn to forgive.** Forgiving someone who has hurt you allows you to move on. Dwelling on others' wrongdoings towards you keeps you in the victim role. Liberate yourself!

What are three things from the ideas above that you could do this week?
What will stop you from being happy today?

Summary

Everything can be taken from a man but one thing: the last of the human freedoms – to choose one's attitude in any given set of circumstances, to choose one's own way.

Viktor E. Frankl, Nazi concentration camp survivor
Man's Search for Meaning (1984)

This chapter has been about starting points. To make a change there has to be awareness that something needs changing, so an evaluation tool like the Wheel of Life is very useful for assessing your satisfaction levels as they are right now. The tool is also useful for measuring your growth of satisfaction in different areas of your life over time. We use it as an annual barometer of how things are going in our lives. It is a quick, visible summary of how satisfied we are in our lives. It is very rewarding seeing the positive correlation between our age, our personal and professional development strategies and satisfaction levels recorded on the wheel each year!

To make changes, we find it is very useful to write down what our plans are and then set goals. For many people, this is enough to make the changes they desire. For others, developing and discussing their plans in a confidential and supportive environment can be the key to successfully making major changes in their life. More people each year are using a coach for this process, and they then commit themselves to scheduling time to explore and plan what will work for them. A coach can also play a strong role in supporting, encouraging and reminding you of the goals you set for yourself and opening up areas for discussion that they feel are appropriate to explore in more depth. Coaching is an option that works well for healthy people as the process can enhance both your professional and personal life, by assisting you in establishing a way of caring for your own well-being. A professional coach provides a partnership, and as coaches, we too have our own coach to ensure that we put the time and energy into our lives as much as we encourage our clients to, so that we genuinely live out the lifestyle we profess to others. The time set aside for coaching appointments provides you with some thinking space, time to truly reflect on where you are and where you want to be, which is a scarce commodity for many health professionals.

Don't wait for a critical incident before you make the changes you know you want in your life. Take action today. It does not matter how small that action may be, the important thing is that you start.

References

Chapman, G. (1995) *The Five Love Languages: How to express heartfelt commitment to your mate.* United States, Northfield Publishing.

Covey, S. (1989) *The 7 Habits of Highly Effective People*. New York, Simon and Schuster.

Firth-Cozens, J. (2003) Doctors, their wellbeing, and their stress. *British Medical Journal*, **326:** 670–671.

Frankl, V. (1984) *Man's Search for Meaning*. New York, Washington Square.

Health & Safety Executive (2004) *Psychosocial Working Conditions in Great Britain in 2005*.

Lyubomirsky S, King L. (2005) The benefits of frequent positive affect: does happiness lead to success? *Psychological Bulletin*, **131**: 803–855.

Smith, A., Brice, C., Collins, A., Mathews, V., McNamara, R. (2000) *The Scale of Occupational Stress: A further analysis of the impact of demographic factors and type of job*. Norwich, HSE Books.

Whitworth, L., Kimsey-House, H., Davies, S. (1998) *Co-active Coaching*, California, Black Publishing.

Values, beliefs and congruency

5

Suzanne Henwood

To be a leader you need to know what is important to you and then make sure all you actions draw you close to that place.

Introduction

Having looked at yourself in greater depth and having begun to think about what you want to change in yourself, you might be left with some questions about 'why'. Why do you want to change those things? Why have those things come to mind as you have worked through those chapters?

This chapter will help you to uncover your core values and beliefs to help to understand why you feel the way you do about your job, about yourself and about your future career progression. One of the most powerful things you can do in terms of self-development and for your own well-being is to bring your values and beliefs into congruency (or alignment) with your behaviours and actions. If any of your core values are being compromised at work, that may well be the cause of any dissatisfaction you are feeling, though you may not have had the tools available to understand why. This chapter will help you to explore your own values and beliefs and the values of your workplace so that you can identify the source of any internal discomfort, thereby giving you the opportunity to resolve that conflict through understanding it and making the appropriate changes.

What are beliefs?

Beliefs are the things we hold true internally, things we have taken on board from significant others, through education, from traumas, from our culture and from life events. Many of our beliefs are formed very early in life and then are reinforced by us in each new situation we find ourselves in. Beliefs shape what we do, and they motivate and drive us. They are not necessarily factually correct, though we often assume they are; indeed when we believe something, we do act as if that belief were true. Beliefs are strongly held emotionally, and people may be prepared to fight for them. Aside from conflicts between cultures and countries, think for a moment about some of the inter-disciplinary conflicts in healthcare, arising from differing beliefs, which have arisen over the years:

- only radiologists can interpret x-rays
- maternity care assistants cannot help deliver babies
- vascular nurses can't strip veins
- midwives can't do ultrasound
- nurses and physiotherapists cannot request x-rays
- nurses can't prescribe medication

I could go on, and I am sure you can think of your own examples, related to your own professional boundaries. These are beliefs which in the past have been fought for and fought over and which, in many cases, have now changed as experience and practices have changed.

As well as core beliefs we all share, like some of the laws of nature, for example that the earth is round (although that was not always a belief held by everyone), or that gravity exists to pull us towards the earth's core, we all also hold beliefs about all sorts of things which are less well defined. For example we hold beliefs about ourselves and our abilities (I am not good enough, I am great at my job) and about others (she doesn't care, he will never amount to anything, he's a leader in the making). We hold beliefs about relationships, difficulties, the way forward and so on. Some beliefs that you might hold as a healthcare practitioner include:

- I believe nurses are generally caring people
- I believe there is always something new to learn
- I believe we should be there to serve patients and their families
- I believe that excellent and open communication is central to great patient care

It might be worth pausing here to consider what beliefs your patients or colleagues may have about you and your service. Just take a moment to jot down a few ideas, maybe think back to how you have felt when you have sought medical attention for yourself. What were your beliefs about the staff? Were they empowering or disempowering? How did those beliefs affect the way you interacted with the staff who treated you? Now just take a few moments and go through that list again and consider how your own actions in practice either confirm or conflict with those same beliefs that patients may also hold about you.

It is worth reflecting on the following question: what effort do you make in order to understand and respect people's beliefs, especially patients; not necessarily agreeing with them, but respecting what is important to them? Do you take time to consider what patients believe about you, about your work, about their treatment, about themselves and their illness even? What difference would it make if you had that information available to you?

The important thing to recognise about beliefs is that they determine how we live our lives. They govern our behaviour. They can act as self-fulfilling, so we prove them over and over to reinforce them, we think and behave in a manner which is in line with our beliefs, we work to maintain them. Think back to the sections on language on p. 56 and on internal dialogue on p. 33 and consider again the power of our language and how that controls our behaviour.

What beliefs do you vocalise internally? A useful question to ask yourself when you hear your internal voice saying something negative or difficult is, 'What has to be true about me for that to be true?' It may be that this reveals some limiting beliefs; if it does, this is excellent material to take to a coach to work through and change.

Another application of beliefs in medicine is the placebo effect. If a patient receives treatment and believes it will work, it will sometimes work even when a placebo has been given in place of the real drug. Conversely, if you prescribe a treatment and alert the patient to the fact that it might not work, you are probably reducing the chances of it working, as the patient will try to confirm that through their reactions to the drug. It is worth considering the power of this with all treatments and drugs, to give wherever possible positive messages about how effective it is expected to be, obviously while paying due attention to actual realistic predictions of possible effectiveness. Think about how best to frame the information for best possible effect on the patients.

Beliefs can also prove to be a stumbling block, preventing us from doing something. You may not even be aware of having such a block, and as we alluded to earlier, a coach can help you to identify and remove such blocks surprisingly easily. For example, if you believe you are not very good at your job, you will behave in such a way as to prove it. You will make mistakes and you will justify them by saying, 'See, I told you I was not very good at my job'. If you say, 'I can't . . .' the chances are you won't. What would happen if instead you thought of the 'can't' as a temporary phase, and added the word 'yet' as we discussed in

Chapter 3? Now that there is a possibility that you might at some point in the future, it makes the achievement possible.

Beliefs operate in this way at a deep level and can override more superficial desires that we are more aware of. It is the belief that determines behaviour, not our conscious thought. One of the best ways to find out the full extent of your capabilities is to pretend or act as if you can do something. Clearly within healthcare you have to take care to act professionally and appropriately and not to put any patient at risk, but how different would your practice be if you acted as if you were excellent at your job, that you were a leader in your field?

One really exciting thing to note from this is that beliefs can be changed. If the beliefs you hold are not generating the results you want in your life and work practice, then work with someone to change them, don't let them hold you back any longer.

Exercise 5.1
Exploring Your Beliefs

Take some time to consider:

- Which beliefs do you hold which are helping you to be who you want to be and which beliefs are holding you back?
- Which beliefs that you hold are helping you to get where you want to get in your career and which are holding you back?
- Which beliefs would help you to be the person you want to be?
- Can you start to act as if those beliefs were already true?
- What difference would that make? What would your life be like?

You choose to believe what you believe. If your beliefs are not supporting you or helping you to be happy and successful, you ought to consider changing them. Do you believe you are (or can be) successful? Believing you are successful is not a guarantee of being successful every time in everything you do. It does, however, leave open the possibility of success and leaves you in a more resourceful state so that you can succeed in some things, some of the time.

It is interesting to note here that our minds cannot distinguish reality from vividly imagined dreams and thoughts. If you start to vividly imagine living with your new beliefs, you will be amazed at how easily and quickly things start to change in your life.

What are values?

So, having spent some time looking at our beliefs, let's spend some time exploring values. Values are closely related to and support our beliefs. Perhaps surprisingly, people may be less aware of the values they hold than they are of their beliefs, even though values relate to their identity. Values are the things that are important to us. They determine how we do something, they determine the direction we travel in, and they motivate and drive us towards our goals. They are the 'fundamental principles we live by' (O'Connor and Seymour, 1995). Values also determine how we feel about something, so if you feel uncomfortable in any given situation it may be that the issue you are considering is in conflict with one or more of your values. For example, values you hold as a healthcare practitioner might include:

- Ongoing Learning
- Trust
- Making a Difference
- Excellence
- Team Work
- Integrity

Of course, each and every one of us will have a different meaning behind each of these words, and on an individual basis it is important to understand what you mean by the words you use to define your values. When exploring your values, it is essential to also ask yourself why that is important to you and how you know whether or not that value is being met in any given context.

Like beliefs, values may change over time and to some extent will differ in different contexts, for example home, work or leisure, or indeed for any of the segments in your Wheel of Life. We tend to retain values that we have chosen to adopt for longer than those that have been imposed on us.

Values at work are an important component of both motivation and job satisfaction. If your values do not match those of your workplace, if they are not congruent, you will not be giving 100% of yourself at work, or worse still you may find yourself in conflict within the workplace, which can then be a very uncomfortable place to be. As a manager it is useful to know whether or not employees' values are being met, since if they are not it might explain why you are not getting a fully committed member of staff, or you are experiencing conflict, high absenteeism or high turnover. Exercise 5.2 later in this chapter is really useful in helping you to identify your values at work and understanding your feelings about your work. It is also a great tool to help you make a decision between two jobs, when considering new options. Set aside half an hour to work through the exercise. You might also consider getting a colleague to help you, as it is sometimes easier to do with someone else asking the questions, and just pushing you a little for answers.

In the workplace values and beliefs are only retained within a department's culture if they are being lived out in practice. This is especially important to remember if you are a manager of a department. If you verbalise that ongoing learning is important to you and within the department, yet you fail to support, encourage or acknowledge ongoing learning, your actions will not be congruent and the sincerity of the value will be open to question by employees. If you say that fun is an important value within the team, yet you do not show that you are having fun yourself, your staff may doubt whether or not fun is really important to you. Figure 5.1 below provides a list of potential values to consider.

Sue Knight (*NLP at Work*, 2002) compares the links between behaviour and values and beliefs to an iceberg (see Figure 5.2). Behaviour is the visible tip, while values, beliefs, purpose, capabilities and identity sit below the surface. They are the internal thoughts and feelings. How often we judge others by the visible tip, the behaviour, without taking time to understand what sits beneath!

Autonomy	Planning
Being Creative	Perfection
Being Encouraged	Potential
Belonging	Progressing
Caring	Qualifications
Commitment	Quality
Communicating	Researching
Education	Sense of Adventure
Empathy	Service
Enjoying	Standards
Excellence	Status
Exciting	Stimulating
Experimenting	Successful
Expertise	Supporting and Being Supported
Fun	Taking Risks
Helping Others	Teaching
Influencing	Team Player
Inspiring	Team Work
Integrity	Time Keeping
Leading	Trust
Learning	Using Imagination
Loyalty	Valued
Making a Difference	Variable
Money	Work/Life Balance
Nurturing	
Ongoing Learning	
Originality	

Figure 5.1   Potential Values (not exhaustive)

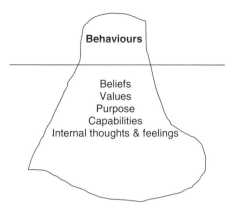

Figure 5.2 The Iceberg Theory

It would be a good use of time as a department to identify your values and beliefs, along with your purpose (why you exist), your vision (what you will look like and be like in the future) and mission (using the definition of how you will work, although it is sometimes used in the same context as purpose). It is wise to be transparent about these issues and ensure that at every point of contact these same values and beliefs are visible, being what Peter Senge called a 'Transparent Department'. If you do not know where you are going or how you are going to get there, you can do nothing more than drift along, hoping that you might be going in the right direction. Why leave it to chance? A little time spent exploring your values and beliefs in relation to your vision and purpose will give you a much greater chance of fulfilling your purpose even more quickly.

Exercise 5.2
Eliciting Values at Work

Sit quietly with a sheet of paper in front of you. Ask yourself the following questions numbered 1 to 5 and then continue by working with your responses.

Alternatively find a colleague and sit and do this for each other. You may find talking it out loud helps you to clarify the points you raise.

1. **'What is important to me in work, my career, my job?'**
   Choose whichever word is most appropriate for you. What do you want from this area of your life?
   This should be answered in the here and now – as work actually is, not as you would like it to be. If you are really stuck, look again at Figure 5.1 for a table of possible values to inspire you.

Write down a list of values that come to mind.
You may have anything from 3 to 10 or even more. Some will be very similar. Don't worry about that now, just write down the values which come to mind.

2. **Ask yourself, 'What else?'**
Just pause and think again, and you might be surprised how easily other values come to mind. Write them down on the bottom of your list.

3. **Ask again, 'What else?'**
Repeat this until no new values emerge.

4. **Think of a time, a specific time, when you were really motivated and enthusiastic about your job. Get a picture of that time in your head. Where were you? What job was it?**

   Now ask yourself, 'What was it about that job that made me really motivated?'
   Add anything new to your list.

5. **Now read down your list and ask yourself, 'If I had all this in a job, what would make me leave?'**
Write down anything new.
   You will now have potentially quite a long list of values.

6. **Read down the list and rank the top eight values.**
   So, which is the most important thing to you? Mark that number 1.
   Which is the second most important thing to you? Mark that number 2.
   Continue until you have marked the top eight.
   If you find it difficult to decide on a single ranking for two values, look only at those two and force yourself to decide. If you could have only one of them, which would it be? Then place that as the higher ranked value.

7. **Write out the new list of eight values on a new sheet of paper, with plenty of space between each value.**

   For each value ask yourself:
   'What has to happen or what has to be present to have . . . ?'
   If you are struggling, look at it in reverse:
   'What would have to be missing for me not to experience . . . ?'

   This list will give you a great indication of where your motivation for your job is coming from, and the origin of any dissatisfaction. This then gives you the information you require to go and obtain that satisfaction by filling those gaps.

I am sure you can see just how useful and valuable this tool can be to help you to look at your own job satisfaction and motivation in a new way. The tool can be used across all the contexts of your Wheel of Life.

Sandra's story below shows how this tool can be used in practice, in this case to assist with a work transition issue.

Sandra's Story

Sandra is a healthcare lecturer who has just returned to work following six months' maternity leave. She is 42 and had almost given up on the thought of having children. She had a difficult end stage of pregnancy and delivery and spent some time on sick leave which extended her maternity period by several weeks.

On return to work Sandra has found it very difficult to leave her daughter, and has felt dissatisfied at work and is finding it difficult to get back any enthusiasm for work.

During her time of absence the organisation she works for underwent a significant change, resulting in her job being very different on return and she is potentially facing redundancy.

Sandra wanted to explore her feelings of dissatisfaction and we suggested using the values model to look at whether her values had changed (Sandra had previously elicited her work values when looking at a promotion opportunity 18 to 24 months previously. She also felt that some of her values were not being met, but she had not spent time specifically identifying those.)

We used the tool described in Exercise 5.2.

So Sandra, what word best describes what you do? Is it work? Your job?

Yes it's my job.

Great. so what is important to you in your job?

Flexibility, that's really important. By that I mean working hours, volume of work, place of work. I want to be able to work at home;

Autonomy, being able to plan what I do;

Responsibility and accountability (they are linked for me);

Not to travel – a local job;

I need colleagues, a team;

Satisfaction;

Useful;

I want it to have some teeth – so I can bring about change, be able to effect change;

A job where I am working for the greater good;

Seniority;

Important, meaningful;

Very well paid. I want more money.

(N.B. after pauses I asked, 'Anything else?' until Sandra could not think of any new values)

So Sandra, can you think of a time when you were really motivated in your job? What was it about that time that motivated you?

I can remember a time (cites a specific meeting). There was a real buzz . . .

What was it that gave that buzz?

Team spirit – group commitment to making it the best;

Excitement about opportunities ahead;

I felt like I was fulfilling my potential;

It felt like we were approaching a special time, there was real group coherence, joined up thinking. We all wanted the same thing;

We were clear and focused;

It felt like the right place, at the right time, with the right people and we were doing the right thing.

Sandra, if you had all of the things on this list, what would make you leave your job?

If travelling became excessive;

If there was disharmony in the group or team;

If the team lost its direction and cohesiveness;

It there was loss of vision or goals.

All of those issues were already covered in her list so I did not at this stage add any new values to my notes.

Sandra, can you look at this list and tell me which is the most important thing to you?

Definitely number 1 would be the meaningful stuff and having a purpose. Then Flexibility would be number 2.

We then discussed Sandra's third, fourth and fifth priorities, grouped some values together under one new descriptive word, and then tested the order and changed it by establishing which one was more important than the next one on the list. The final list became:

1. *'Change' – this incorporated being able to effect change, having responsibility and accountability, and it also included seniority.*
2. *Autonomy – though this could be linked to flexibility.*
3. *'Cohesiveness' – this incorporated group dissonance, team spirit, etc.*
4. *Well paid. More money.*
5. *Excitement about opportunities ahead.*

Sandra was not sure if number 5 was the value, and in talking we determined that the value was about fulfilling her potential, which gave her excitement as a result.

> Sandra, let's compare that with your values hierarchy for work previously, before you became pregnant. What has changed?

> *Flexibility is the only real change – it has gone way higher up.*

> And at present you have that flexibility, so it is not that which is generating your dissatisfaction. Have a look and see if you can identify what is missing.

> *(Laughing) It's that top one. It's not about the baby! It's the changes at work. I haven't got a sense of purpose any more. There's nothing competing with my purpose of being a mother, so that has pride of place, that's why I don't want to come in to work. There's no balance, and I don't want there to be a balance – because of the situation at work.*

> Sandra, what has to be present for there to be a sense of purpose?

> *There needs to be a clear purpose – clear objectives – I don't have that any more.*

> How would you know if you did have it?

> *It would be a strong feeling. A core feeling of warmth within me, I would know all the value boxes had been ticked, I would know my job was important, that it was needed by the greater world, that I was valued.*

> Sandra then realised that if the job had remained intact and all courses had
> still been up and running, she would not have felt so reluctant to go to work.
> She felt that:
>
> *I'm feeling a sense of purposelessness.*
>
> *If I was contributing to society, then that's as important as being a mum,
> you need to feel you are doing something useful outside the house. This
> is not just about leaving the baby, it's a transition, being a working woman
> with a purpose, only I haven't got one here in this job.*

Undertaking this exercise showed Sandra what the issue was that was causing dissatisfaction, and left her with options, as she now knows what she needs to tackle to resolve it. Alternatively, she can decide if it is time to move on if she feels that she is not going to achieve a sense of purpose in her job. Before undertaking this exercise Sandra was convinced her dissatisfaction was related to her new status as a mother. The tool gave her clarity about the real cause of her dissatisfaction.

Values and decision making

Eliciting values is also a great way to help you to make a decision about a new job, or new work opportunity. Using the tool in Exercise 5.2 on page 87, elicit the values for work and then compare that list against the values of the job options you are considering. You can then score each value from your list out of ten for each job option and then give an overall score for each job being considered, or compare the score of your current job with a proposed new job or promotion. You will find a table on the accompanying website www.wiley.com/go/nlphealthcare to help you in this exercises.

You might find you cannot score some of the values, as you do not know the answer. This then gives you great questions to ask in a preliminary phone call or during an interview. If you know ongoing learning is important to you, ensure you ask about the development opportunities and support available in the new job, before you accept it. If you know that you enjoy working in a team, ask about the structure of the department and what opportunity you will have to contribute to that team. You can even ask for the values of the new department to see if there is any conflict with your own. Of course, always look for evidence that these values are being actively played out in the department, and be aware that some departments may not be able to tell you what their values are as they may not have thought about their department in this way. Do not rely solely on a verbalised report of what someone thinks the values should be, ask other staff about those issues during your visit.

Values, beliefs and conflict – finding congruency

We spoke earlier in the book about the Communication Model. Associated with this is the phrase: 'The Map is not the Territory' (see Chapters 2 and 5). When two people, with different maps, create different meanings (internal representations) from an event or a situation, there is a real potential for conflict. Values and Beliefs form a central part of your Map of the Territory, or your Map of Reality. If we start to impose our map on other people and we start to insist that what we find important should also be important to them, we are not respecting their map or their reality. This does not mean you have to agree with the other's point of view, but it does mean that you should work to recognise that other views exist, and that you should attempt to understand the other view and recognise any imposition of your views onto others.

Conflict does not just exist between two people. You can also experience internal conflict or incongruence. Let's consider for example a nurse who has a list of tasks to do which is too long to accomplish in the time available to her. The nurse, an avid NLP supporter, knows and understands her values at work, one of which is to maintain high standards of patient care. As she is walking towards a patient to change a dressing, another patient, an elderly man, confined to bed, vomits over himself and his bed. She knows she is alone on that bay of patients and has no one else to call on for at least half an hour. She has a duty of care to both patients. She also has a number of choices, some of which include:

- Option 1 – Pretend she did not notice and keep walking (the patient has not called out to her).
- Option 2 – Acknowledge the problem and keep on walking, explaining to the patient that she is in the middle of something and will get back to him as soon as possible.
- Option 3 – Stop what she is doing and clean the patient and advise him she will be back to sort the bed in due course.
- Option 4 – Stop what she is doing and clean the patient, change the bedding and ensure he is comfortable.
- Option 5 – Stop what she is doing, clean the patient up, change the bedding, ensure he is comfortable and explore why he had vomited and record the information in the patient's notes, whilst ensuring that the other patient is aware of the reason for the delay in their dressing being changed.

Options 1 and 2 are so greatly in conflict with her values of high standards of patient care that they can be quickly dismissed as an option. She would not be comfortable walking past and not responding, even though she is all cleaned up and ready to change a dressing on another patient and is indeed carrying the tray of supplies required.

Option 3 is a possibility. This will depend on the position of the value in the hierarchy and what constitutes high standards of patient care to the nurse.

Option 4 is also a possibility and is likely to be the outcome for those who place high standards of patient care in the top four values of their work.

Option 5 will be selected by those who place high standards of patient care in the top spot of values at work.

This is of course all assuming that the other patient is safe and can wait to have her dressing changed.

What is important to note is that it is a conflict internally between your own values and your proposed behaviour (of walking past the patient) that gives you the uncomfortable feeling. Recognising this incongruence is a valuable skill and through practice of heightening your awareness of the feelings associated with both congruency and incongruency in yourself, you can learn to ensure that you remain true to your values and beliefs, which will give you personal strength, courage and power to act appropriately.

Other potential sources of internal incongruence in healthcare professionals may include:

- Would you withhold information from a patient if you thought it was in their best interests?
- Would you cover up a clinical error for a colleague to cover their back?
- Would you apply for a tedious job if it was close to home and offered a perceived better quality of life by reducing the hours away from home each day?

So how do we know when we are internally congruent or incongruent?

For many it will be an internal feeling that will indicate whether or not they feel comfortable with a decision they have made or an action they have taken. Look at both what you say and what you do. Are the two in alignment? Look beyond yourself and look at whether or not you are congruent within your workplace, or more widely still, within your profession?

Once you have established that you are congruent, you will have available to you all your inner resources and you are likely to be more highly motivated to achieve success.

Wider alignment?

Once you start to look at internal congruence and then your own 'fit' within a department in relation to your values, you are operating at a deeper level than you have probably done before. I am now going to push you one more level and get you to look at Alignment, using a model based on the one developed by Robert Dilts called 'Neurological Levels of Change'.

Dilts presented his model as a hierarchy, a pyramid of six levels of change. We prefer to think of the model as interconnected issues which all impact on and interrelate, demonstrating that by changing one you are likely to impact on another. It is nonetheless a useful model for exploring the different components of change that you need to consider.

In fact this is a great tool to use in relation to any aspect of change when you are thinking about yourself, about your team or department, or even about your employers, be they a hospital, Trust, private company or group of independent practitioners.

The components of change are:

- environment
- behaviour
- capabilities
- beliefs and values
- identity
- purpose

A good way to explore this is to look at the statement:

'I can't do that here'

If someone says this, listen to the emphasis on each word. The tone and emphasis on particular words will indicate what level or component of change is a concern or issue.

For example, I can't do that *here*, would indicate an issue of environment. You might explore:

'Where can't you do it?'

'When can't you do it?'

'With whom can't you do it?'

Compare this to: I can't do *that* here, which would alert you to issues of behaviour. An appropriate question may then be:

'What is it you cannot do?'

Or alternatively: I can't *do* that here, which would point to capability. This would lead you to ask questions about how something was being done.

Once the emphasis moves to I *can't* do that here, you are moving to the 'values and beliefs' level in the model by Dilts, and you would be asking,

'Why can't that be done?'

If the emphasis is on *I* can't do that here, the issue lies more deeply, with issues of identity or potentially also purpose. Who is it that cannot do something and why is something not being done?

The hierarchical model is useful because it helps you realise that if the issue is one of values or beliefs, then changing the environment, or providing training to ensure capability, is not going to solve the problem. Instead, you have to operate at least one level above where the issue rests. This can be useful, but is too simplistic to cover all aspects related to these components of change, and while it is worth considering, you have to consider all components and the relationship between the components to really understand change. It is important to be aware of the different components and understand how changing one will impact or not on others to ensure you work with someone on the right issue to achieve the desired outcome. In terms of congruence it is important to ensure that all levels are in alignment and support each other for the best possible outcomes.

Considering this in relation to a healthcare department – let's take for example a ward context. Think of what happens when a new ward manager is appointed and wishes to install a new culture of quality and patient centredness. If that manager works with staff on their behaviour, Dilts would argue that their beliefs are not going to be affected and consequently the change may be superficial or short lived. In order to ensure that the change in culture is permanent and fully embedded, work would also have to be done on values and beliefs; employing a coach could enable you to do this for individuals within the team and for the team as a whole. We could argue that by changing staff behaviours there might be a knock-on effect on their beliefs as experience redefines the belief in the light of the new behaviour and the outcome it generates. Why leave this to chance, being aware that work on values and beliefs is also required? Now that you understand the different components of change you could work on those values to ensure the change is embedded. When looking at appropriate development for this kind of work, you might want to consider when skills training is required and when deeper work on values and beliefs is essential.

Another point to consider, raised by Knight (2002), is that by focusing on the environment and capabilities, it means that we focus on our and others' behaviours in the work environment. We will then notice and react to changes in behaviour, making us more reactive in our approach. If we are more reactive we are less likely to be leading from the front and forging our own direction for the future. If we can switch our attention away from environment and abilities, to issues of values, beliefs, identity and purpose, we can work more independently and truly be leaders in our field.

How is this all relevant in a chapter on values and beliefs? For me, it comes back to the issue of congruence. Take time to consider yourself in the light of each of the levels or components of change. Consider how things are in each component and also how you would like them to be. Just take a moment to explore the various levels using Exercise 5.3.

Exercise 5.3
Logical Levels of Change

It is a good idea to have someone with you to ask you the questions and to take notes of your thoughts so you can refer back to them afterwards.

Consider the role that you have (staff nurse, physiotherapist, manager, leader, researcher, lecturer, etc.). Take five sheets of blank paper and write one of these words on each sheet:

Environment

Capability / Behaviour

Values / Beliefs

Identity

Purpose

Place the pieces of paper across the floor in a straight line, in the order they appear in the list above.

Stand firstly on the paper marked 'Environment' and ask (or have a colleague ask you):

Where are you a . . . ? (insert here your role / title)

Where else?

When are you a . . . ?

Move on to Capability / Behaviour and ask:

What do you do as a . . . ?

What are you good at as a . . . ?

What are you less good at as a . . . ?

Move on to Values / Beliefs and ask:

> What is important to you as a . . . ?
>
> What do you believe as a . . . ?

Move on to Identity. Really feel what it is like to be a . . . and ask:

> Who are you as a . . . ?
>
> What labels would you put on yourself as a . . . ?
>
> How would someone else describe you as a . . . ?
>
> If you had everything you desired as a . . . who would you be?

Move on to Purpose and ask:

> Why are you a . . . ?
>
> What are you trying to achieve as a . . . ?

At any stage you can ask, 'What else?' to gain even more information.
   Once you have travelled from one end of the line to the other, turn round and walk back down that line in reverse.

> Move back to Identity and ask:
>
> > Who would you like to be as a . . . ?
>
> Step back to Values / Beliefs and ask:
>
> Bringing that new sense of self with you, what is important to you now as a . . . ?
>
> Step back to Capability / Behaviour and ask:
>
> > What do you need to develop as a . . . ?
>
> Step back to Environment and ask:
>
> > Where else could you be a great . . . ?
> >
> > When else could you be a great . . . ?

Step off the paper and stand back so you can see all the sheets on the floor. Just take a few moments to consider:

> What insights did you have during this process?
>
> What else did you notice?
>
> How does this affect your motivation as a . . . ?
>
> What are you going to do now?

This is a very useful tool and Jean's story illustrates just how it was used to demonstrate incongruence in her professional life.

Jean's Story

Jean is a manager and is experiencing some difficulties with a small group of staff. She felt she had tried everything to resolve those difficulties and was now experiencing frustration at her own apparent inability to influence things in her department.

Jean walked through the logical levels model and on the way back down when she stood on Capabilities / Behaviour, she realised that her behaviour was not congruent with her values. In particular she recognised she was being too controlling, not trusting her staff to handle the situation and she was being too quick to jump in and make suggestions, which was only exacerbating the situation.

Jean had a real emotional reaction at this point in the exercise and when she stood away from the paper sheets she was able to identify new choices in how to handle the difficulties she was presented with and returned to work feeling re-energised and able to cope.

Despite Jean having 'tried everything', which was her perception, this tool enabled her to gain a new perspective and revealed the cause of her discomfort, which then opened up new choices to her which she could apply to resolve the issue with her staff.

Summary

In this chapter we have explored values and beliefs and looked at ways of raising our awareness in both areas. We have also looked at the importance of ensuring that our values and beliefs are being met at work in order to ensure a high level of personal satisfaction and motivation. It may be that in exploring issues at this depth you actually come to the realisation that a core value is not being met at work and you can now tackle how to change that. It may be of course that you recognise that the value cannot be met at your current workplace and actually it would be better to move on.

The tools are in one respect quite simple and they are also incredibly powerful. Use them to get to know and understand yourself even more. Explore all possibilities and understand fully the contribution you can and do make. You may be surprised just how easily you become aware of other options and new routes. Just because you cannot see any light coming through a doorway, do not automatically assume the doorway does not exist.

References

Dilts, R. (1990) *Changing Belief Systems with NLP*. London, Meta Publications.
Knight, S. (2002) *NLP at Work: The difference that makes a difference in business*. London, Nicholas Brealey Publishing.
O'Connor, J. and Seymour, J. (1995) *Introducing NLP: Psychological skills for understanding and influencing people*. London, Thorsons.
Senge, P. (1994) *The Fifth Discipline: The art and practice of the learning organisation*. London, Currency Doubleday.

Perceptual positioning

6

Jim Lister

Can we ever truly understand another person's perspective until we have tried walking in their shoes for a while?

In Chapter 2 we introduced you to the Communication Model which emphasised the unique 'map' each of us has internally about what occurs externally. We shared with you how that map is formed and what variations to be aware of in different interpretations of events. We also explored the issue of self-empowerment and followed that in Chapter 3 by looking at how we can empower ourselves to others, how we can change people's perceptions of us. We then explored in greater depth our inner values and beliefs which determine behaviour, to help us to understand some of the 'why' behind the differences we experience with others and also internally when we feel at conflict with situations around us. Can we safely assume that from here on there will be no more conflict, no more difficulties? Pretty unlikely. Despite knowing why we are in conflict with someone and despite understanding our own inner motivations better, we are still likely from time to time to find ourselves in a situation which we find uncomfortable or stressful. Wouldn't it be great to have a tool to tackle such conflict and difference of opinion, in a positive and structured way to ensure respect is shown to both parties? In fact could you imagine becoming so familiar with such a tool that you start to employ it even before the conflict escalates into a real situation which needs to be resolved? Well, the good news is that is exactly what we present here: a tool to help you resolve conflict, which when you are familiar with it, can be used across a variety of different settings, making it possibly the most flexible and useful tool we present in this book.

Embracing diversity

You will by now appreciate the extent to which this book emphasises the need to respect the unique make-up and distinctive identity of each individual, both your-self and those you meet. You must also inevitably be aware of how the social and geographical mobility of the modern world has created a culturally rich and varied workforce. You only need to look around at your colleagues and your patients to appreciate the remarkable multicultural diversity of 21st-century life. This developing trend of diversity, and the accompanying need to pay due regard to each individual's unique character and identity, presents us with great oppor-tunities and numerous demanding but exciting challenges.

Rather than interpreting this as a threat to familiar values, loaded with intractable problems and latent conflict, it is of course infinitely more constructive to view global multicultural diversity as an engrossing opportunity for social enrichment and productive human interaction. As Augustus Casely-Hayford observes in his article entitled 'We all need to change our ways' in *The Independent* on August 23 2006, 'the underpinning narrative and values of contemporary Britain have subtly, but profoundly, altered'. He elaborates further:

> The idea of a stable mainstream founded upon a fixed core set of ideals and beliefs against which everything else is measured and accommodated, must be seen as an old-fashioned comforting delusion. I hope that we now accept that our society is and always has been much more complex. Embracing, not just accommodating, that complexity has to be part of our future – we almost have no choice.

This urgent need to expand the horizons of our thinking affects us not only in our day-to-day interactions as individuals, but also in the broader perspectives we choose to adopt with regard to rapidly changing local, national and global condi-tions. The onus is therefore on us to explore and refine fresher and more flexible patterns of thinking, liberating us from the outmoded, rigid range of reactions we have inherited from social and cultural conditions lately superseded by diverse and complex new realities. NLP offers practical strategies for nurturing and exploring just the kinds of imaginative, experimental and empathetic channels of thought that will be crucial if we are to negotiate the at times bewildering diversity of expe-riences with which we are now confronted. This is particularly useful in healthcare because of the stresses unique to the profession, such as patient vulnerability.

Implications for the workplace

This chapter therefore deals with a key question raised by these issues: how do we adapt to and embrace the complex challenges presented by this developing cultural (in its widest sense) diversity in our workplace? Healthcare is a people-based service, consisting of huge numbers of employees at all levels. The focus of our work in healthcare is effective patient care. People obviously form the fundamental resource and purpose of the service. However, people can at times seem to us to be such an obstacle to efficiency! I have heard many healthcare colleagues joke that everything would be much more straightforward if only there weren't patients to complicate things. I have also often heard the observation that 'things would be fine if only I ran things and worked with patients – it's the staff and my colleagues who get in the way!'

So wherever we have people, working under the increasingly stressful, pressurised, under-resourced conditions that now characterise healthcare provision, there is inevitably, in my experience, a degree of anxiety, uncertainty, tension and conflict which seems to bear down on employees and affect healthy working relationships. How does this day-to-day pressure manifest itself inside you? Do you recognise it? How do you manage it? How do you influence and persuade the other person or the team who seem to block your good ideas? It would be great to work in an environment where everyone agreed, people deferred to each other and conducted themselves in an overwhelming spirit of cooperation. And where pigs might, and do, fly . . .

The map is not the territory

Our reality is of course very different, and it is the word 'difference' that I believe holds a vital clue. As the phrase 'the map is not the territory' clearly illustrates, our own truth is simply our unique interpretation of any event that we experience. This is our internal representation in the Communication Model. Today might seem overpoweringly hot and energy draining to me, but to you it could be uplifting, warming and energising, especially if it is your last day for two weeks as you fly to the Spanish coast on Sunday morning! Another person has their version, and another theirs, and so on.

Before we know it, one simple situation can be viewed from many different maps, not necessarily with any overlap or common ground. We could find that our maps are miles apart, particularly where we hold an impassioned opinion that we believe to be the right way. The other person or team will almost certainly have their own right way. We could even believe that we hold the same map, yet on deeper exploration of what something means to us and to the other person, we may be miles apart. This might help to explain a conflict or difference of opinion you have experienced in the past, which apparently came out of nowhere.

This useful concept of the map, drawn from NLP thinking, was first suggested after considering the London Underground design on the back of the A-Z. It is simply a map and not the territory of London, which is of course far more sophisticated and complex.

Exercise 6.1
Getting to the Meaning

This exercise will help to illustrate the surprising diversity of individual interpretations of even the most commonplace experiences.

Get a group of your colleagues together and provide each with a piece of paper with Figure 6.1 printed in the middle of it.

Each person should, on the circular diagram, write any words that they associate with chocolate. This should be eight single words, one on each spoke; no phrases, just single words, whatever they might be. Don't think too hard, just write the first words that occur to you!

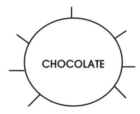

Figure 6.1   Getting to the meaning

Now compare your words to those written by your colleague(s), and discover how few of your words are shared. I have used this exercise hundreds of times with all sorts of different groups, and the same pattern emerges every time – minimal commonality.

So, having explored a simple concept like 'chocolate' and recognised the trend towards difference and diversity, consider how this principle relates to more complex professional issues such as 'personal reviews', 'changing working hours', 'teamwork', 'quality', 'equality' and 'organisational restructure'. No wonder our professional life is prone to frequent poor communication and, at times, a lack of common consensus. The challenge is to control and manage each situation to improve communication and to increase mutual understanding. These goals can be achieved using techniques that we are about to explore, starting with a visual summary of the concept of the perception gap.

'THE MAP IS NOT THE TERRITORY'

My Map or Perception	GAP	Others' Perception or Map
	Beliefs	
	Experiences	
	Cultures	
	States	

Figure 6.2 The map is not the territory

Chapter 2 examined the influences that contribute to our unique identity, our upbringing, value, beliefs and past experiences. This process was encapsulated in the Communication Model. We bring all of our influences to every new experience, and we interpret each experience through the most influential filter of all, our perceptions. We then take our unique interpretations to other people and compare and contrast them. As we have already discovered, we notice immediate differences between our own truths and other people's perceptions of the truth.

So, how do we usually deal with these differences, these perception gaps? There tend to be four options:

* A shared perception/interpretation
* A changing of map or maps
* Agreeing to differ
* No change, or a stand-off

Which of these outcomes do you recognise from your own experience? We have varying degrees of success in managing and resolving situations in which a significant perception gap occurs. Some might argue that we become more effective in managing these difficulties the older and more experienced we become. Others might argue it is the other way round. Sometimes we can utilise a greater level of natural ability, or we can bolster our skills through training. Alternatively we can bring in specialists as third parties to present an independent view to negotiate or mediate on our behalf. We then already have a number of existing coping strategies that offer us support in managing difference and bridging perception gaps which occur between us and other people.

However, these existing coping strategies can seem like mere damage limitation. Might it not be more beneficial and constructive to prepare for the inevitable before it happens? Is it not indeed inevitable, especially in the culturally complex world outlined at the opening of the chapter, that we will at some stage become involved in various types of miscommunication, perception gaps, maps of the territory not coming together, heated debate, and at worst, open conflict? One result of all of this of course is stress, taking us further away from being the effective person we wish to be. We therefore need to become adept at using strategies that will help us forestall these problems before they become destructive. If you have or are experiencing such stress, you might like to work through Chapter 8 before continuing with this one.

Exercise 6.2
Exploring Perception Gaps

This exercise will prepare the way for these 'forestalling strategies' by helping you to reflect on how you have habitually dealt with 'perception gaps' in the past and help you to put in place an even more effective way of dealing with them in the future.

Write down an example of where a 'perception gap' has occurred in your working life. Ask yourself these five questions: notice, and note down, what you notice.

1. What were the different Maps of the Territory?
2. How did you try and deal with the situation?
3. What was the outcome?
4. How long did the process last (and how long did you spend on each step)?
5. Were you satisfied? Was the other party satisfied?

Learning to step back

In the previous exercise, you might have noticed how little time you gave yourself to 'step back' from the heat of the situation, in order to reflect or distance yourself. This is a common trait when we are faced with different maps or conflict, because one of the consequences of being 'in dispute' or at odds with another person is that we often become highly emotionally engaged. A potent cocktail of primary emotional responses kicks in and we find ourselves feeling angry by degree, threatened, unhappy and fearful. Our pride is also inflamed, and we can suddenly find ourselves in the grip of impulses that seem well beyond our control.

You will probably have had experiences in which a problem seems so insurmountable that it is with you morning, noon and night, and even in sleep! There seems no solution no matter what you have tried, it dominates your thoughts, and you feel stressed, and well and truly stuck! The only way of stepping back is to retreat and bury your head in the sand. As you will have found, this whole cycle is demoralising and destructive.

Should someone come along and suggest you take time out, reflect, step back and 'think outside the box', you might hear yourself outwardly, or at the very least inwardly, screaming, 'I've tried. I can't and I haven't the time! I've tried everything!' Well, the questions have to be asked, 'Have you? Is there another way? And how healthy is it for you to carry on this way? How can you step back and usefully reflect?' Acknowledging a perception gap offers a solution that gives you that space to reflect, and brings a different, much more constructive perspective.

Have a look now at Neil's story. An NHS manager, Neil was experiencing all these difficulties, the conflict, the stress, the sleepless nights, but he used his training in the concept of perception gaps to comprehensively overcome the problem.

Neil's Story

For a number of months, we had been trying to attract a consultant to the service I was managing within the Regional Trust. For a variety of reasons, we were having difficulty recruiting for the position, and it was starting to give the impression that the post, and by implication the Trust, was somehow unattractive.

I was serving on a steering group with two consultants from adjacent Trusts in the region. One of the consultants suggested solving the problem by advertising the post in his Trust, by implication a more attractive proposition, and then seconding the consultant to my service through a system linking staff between Trusts.

Whilst this might have offered a feasible solution, I felt that I was being sidelined, and that my influence over my own Trust was being challenged. I had started off in a nursing background, and after seven years working for the Trust, I felt a strong personal responsibility to protect its interests. I feared that if we conceded some control over this issue, it might have a knock-on effect with regard to other initiatives, with the partnership Trust using this consultant recruitment issue as leverage to gain increased influence in other matters of policy. Although I knew and liked the consultant on the steering group who made the suggestion, and we were on good terms, I suspected that personal career advancement might have been behind his offer, and I was uneasy about the prospect of having an employee within my service ultimately being managed by another Trust.

Because of these reservations, I persistently blocked the suggestion within the steering group, and we continued to make no progress in the recruitment of the consultant. Then, following a session with a coach who was working with my Trust, I began to realise that my own narrow perception of the situation was perhaps responsible for the impasse we had reached. Casting round for an alternative interpretation, I applied the 'best intention' principle to the consultant's motives, and acknowledged that ambition, and a bid for increased personal influence, might not have been his dominant motivations at all. I began to appreciate that a concern for the effectiveness of patient care in the whole regional service could very well have been behind the initiative he was suggesting.

The simmering tension that had been starting to erode the effectiveness of the steering group had been caused by a perception gap. I had been defensive and suspicious, adopting an interpretation of events that assumed that my role was being undermined. The consultant's perception was simply that the problem had to be overcome in order to provide a robust medical team, thereby safeguarding the quality of local patient care. Once I had accepted this less sinister motive, the group began operating again in a constructive and open way.

On reflection, a combination of motives might well have been behind the consultant's suggestion. But the point is that by recognising the perception gap, and applying the 'best intention' principle, a sense of reconciliation and collective purpose was re-established. And as often happens when you make concessions to defuse conflict, fate seemed to intervene for the better, almost of its own accord, and I successfully recruited a consultant for my service shortly afterwards.

Reframing an event

Neil's experience reveals the liberating effects of acknowledging a perception gap, and stepping back from a situation to consider conflicting points of view more coolly and objectively. Neil also employed a technique called reframing to overcome this potentially damaging conflict of wills. Reframing means putting another possible meaning on an event, or on someone's motives for acting in a particular way, again demonstrating the powerful effect of using appropriate language as outlined in Chapter 3.

We can approach the technique of reframing by considering an issue that you are dealing with in your working life. Think of a problem that is complex and causing some degree of distress to you. How does it affect you at the moment? How does it make you feel? What have you tried to do about it? Wouldn't it be great if your mind could find a new way of approaching the problem so that it could float away and leave you untroubled, at least until you are able to do something practical about it? Try now to reframe it. We do it all the time anyway, so let's look at it as a conscious process over which we can exert complete control.

Reframing refers to our ability to reinterpret an event or a response for ourselves, in order for us to remain more resourceful and able to progress. It requires us to restrain our initial, instinctive interpretation of an event, or of someone's motives, and search out an alternative, fuller, and perhaps more generous and less suspicious, explanation. It allows us to see something not as a problem but as a 'solution opportunity', a challenge which requires an answer. Having arrived at this reinterpretation, we have gained some breathing space, and we have overridden any potentially destructive temptation to over-react to or misconstrue an event or incident.

Exercise 6.3
Reframing

Reframing is not a particularly complicated or specialised process. You will inevitably have performed it many times, probably without being aware of it. Think of an occasion when you have reframed an event in your life. What happened in your reframing? What were the consequences of the reframing?

You might, for example, have been caught in a long traffic jam in which the traffic was virtually stationary. Your first impulses might have been frustration and impatience, but having realised that the jam was unavoidable, you used the time to calm down and clear your mind, creating a buffer zone from your home and work commitments, used the time to reflect on an issue, time you wouldn't otherwise have spent on it, or took time just to 'chill out', perhaps by listening to some relaxing music. It seems so easy doesn't it? The trick is to gain this vital breathing space by using reframing consciously and consistently, so that it becomes an easy and comfortable process, almost a reflex.

As well as being an exceptionally useful aid in negotiating the everyday demands of being a healthcare professional, reframing can also be immensely helpful during discussion and counselling with patients, and the relatives of patients. Here are the thoughts of Rachel, an experienced NLP practitioner, and a qualified nurse who has also worked as a lecturer and counsellor.

Rachel's Story

Reframing techniques have always been central to my work in healthcare. For example, following appropriate assessment, I might gently try to encourage a shift of perspective in patients who appear to be in denial, perhaps about symptoms or a course of treatment. Without actually using the term 'reframing', I encourage people to modify, or build on, their first reactions by asking questions such as, 'What if things were different to what you now assume, what if this turned out to be the case instead? How would you like things to be if there were a different explanation?' Using these kinds of prompts and suggestions, patients can be encouraged to face up to their situation, while gaining reassurance about the broader range of possible explanations and outcomes. The very act of reflecting on alternatives, seeing the wider perspective, can itself prove to be a calming and therapeutic process whilst often facilitating behavioural shifts.

Often by changing the words we use, we can change our internal representation of the issue, which as we know impacts on our 'state', how we feel, and our behaviour (see the Communication Model in Chapter 2). Play with the words and descriptions you use to see which ones reduce any negative feelings. Be creative about how you describe things and you will be amazed at just what an impact this has.

Moving on from reframing: the next stage

We can therefore use reframing as a helpful first step in confronting issues which appear difficult or are interpreted as distressing challenges. In addition to this process, there are those notably problematic circumstances that affect us especially deeply and consistently unsettle us. These intransigent situations keep coming back at us no matter how much time and effort we give them, eventually seeming all-consuming and insoluble.

As a first step towards finding a strategy for this sort of problem, think of an aspect of your life which isn't going as well as you might have hoped, and despite reframing, is still unresolved and causing you some degree of pain, anxiety, uncertainty or stress. Your example should involve another person, and be a relatively low-key issue. At least at this stage, don't make it the big one! We will be exploring practical ways of dealing with this bigger issue shortly. It is important not to use this for traumatic events – see footnote on p. 122.

Perceptual positioning

The technique of perceptual positioning is a highly effective way of reframing more complex, unresolved and deeply stressful events. It is a hugely powerful thinking tool, a way even of looking at how we live our lives. How many times in education could we have used a technique to enable us to consider how we think, not just what to think? Here is such a tool, credited to John Grinder and Judith De Lozier.

Perceptual positioning is rooted in conflict-resolution strategies. Grinder and De Lozier studied high-achieving people dealing professionally in conflict resolution, from the global to the local, and determined that these people were often using the same thinking strategy although without consciously realising it. They developed the 'three sphere thinking tool' (now known as perceptual positioning), and it works as follows.

By standing in all three positions we will be able to seek positive intentions, and this information will affect our perceptions of the difficulty facing us, which is adversely affecting how we feel.

We can and do choose to place ourselves in any of these three positions at any time within a dialogue with ourselves and/or another person. You may recognise you have a preferred position and you may need to practise standing in the other positions, to be even more proficient at all three positions over time. With practice, you will be surprised just how easily you can move between positions and how this will change how you perceive issues in your life.

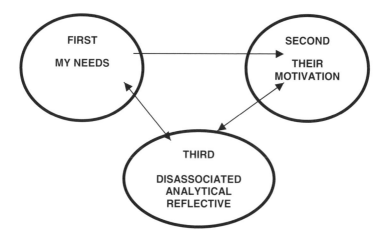

Figure 6.3   Perceptual positioning

First – Looking exclusively subjectively, as I, me, from my experience (the term we use for this is 'associated'). As if looking through your own eyes.

Second – As if I am the other person, looking at them or me (associated: looking as if through their eyes).

Third – Outside of both, looking in, at a distance, the overview (disassociated). This is often referred to as the 'Helicopter View' in management texts. It is where you can see both people in the picture.

Travelling around from position one, to position two, to position three, prevents us becoming trapped in any one 'bubble' and enhances the quality of information available to us to make our decisions. This is especially useful in understanding the motivation of another person whose behaviour is causing us to feel demoralised and stressed.

Perceptual positioning enables us to step back, reflect and understand a situation more fully. It is an incredibly flexible tool which can be used for example in self-coaching and in working with another person, also in decision making and inter-team working. It can be helpful in preparing a presentation, using position two, or a number of different position twos, to represent the different groups of people expected to be in the audience. It is a discipline with a rigorous format that cannot be compromised. However, once the tool is more familiar it is feasible to introduce some flexibility, for example, to return to position two in order to acquire more learning. Initially at least the tool should be followed step by step, and it asks us to look both inwardly and outwardly, distinguishing clearly between cause and effect, to find ways that we can improve any situation for ourselves and for other parties who are involved. It is a highly respectful tool, one that seeks gains for all parties. It is not a technique used to bring someone else down or to gain selfish benefits at the expense of another party. It is a de-stressor, a healthy thinking tonic for all parties involved.

Exercise 6.4
Perceptual Positioning

Here is our version of how to employ perceptual positioning in practice. It has been fine-tuned through working with many case studies in both training and coaching situations. Our evidence tells us it works in this format. Please try this exercise and notice the difference for yourself. Work with a partner, someone you are close to and trust. Their role is simply to ask you the questions at each stage. This exercise should be content free. In other words, you do not have to answer any of the questions aloud, simply to yourself through your own internal dialogue. Do not describe any detail to another person who may be working with you as your 'coach'. Their role is to ask you the questions and to give you the space to respond inwardly to yourself, allowing appropriate amounts of time. This distance between coach and client is vital. The detail of the situation only detracts from the process.

Set up three 'thinking areas' as indicated in Figure 6.3. These could be chairs, or positions marked out on the floor. I suggest that at first you carry out the exercise standing, as this will provide greater energy and will improve the flow of oxygen to the brain. The obvious movement between positions is also helpful to enable you to physically step into the other person's shoes.

Take the example that you considered earlier of a moderate sized problem that has resisted straightforward reframing and keeps coming back to you. As you consider the issue, it will probably create some degree of discomfort in your body and mind. Be aware of this as you work through the following format, a five-step process designed to achieve effective, enduring reframing through the use of 'Perceptual Positioning'.

Prepare yourself for the exercise by asking the following three questions:

- Do I want to resolve this issue?
- Is it OK for me and for others involved to resolve this issue?
- Am I willing to do whatever it takes to resolve this issue?

If the answer to any of these is 'No' you should consider exploring this before proceeding to ensure maximum impact.

STEP 1
Ask yourself the following questions:

1. Who is the other person involved in your problem/issue/predicament?
2. Where are you when this situation typically occurs?
3. When did it first happen and how long has this been running?
4. What are your best intentions for the situation and everyone involved?
5. What do you feel now about the situation and your responses to it so far?

The result of these questions is to become associated with the problem, almost as if it is happening now and the other person or party is present. You will notice some physical reactions, and you may feel injustices, uncertainties and anger to some extent. When you are fully associated and clear about your position here, recognising your actions and beliefs, and your positive intentions, move on to position two. Don't stay too long in one, as this is a position you are already familiar with. If you linger here, and become too emotionally involved, it might prove difficult to move into position two.

STEP 2
Leave position one and 'break state' with the associated feelings by becoming yourself, standing almost in neutral. Think about what you had to eat most

recently or some other useful distraction to take you out of position one. Now take yourself to the second position, in the shoes of the other person, and feel what it might be like to be them. Completely forget yourself, and try to become them as much as possible. Think about how they stand or sit and as much as possible become them. Now, look across to position one and see yourself. You are no longer being you in the situation, because you are seeing it wholly from their point of view. Consider standing as they would stand and as much as possible, get into their shoes, and when you are ready and are beginning to associate with their situation answer these questions to yourself:

1. What is this person feeling about the situation? Dig as deeply as possible.

2. When you now look back at position one, how does person one (you) appear to them?

3. What are their best intentions in all their actions and behaviours?

The result of these questions is to become associated in their world. Through this exploration, huge learning is achieved for ourselves about them and about us and how we have perceived them in the past. When you feel that you have found out as much as you can about their world and how they see you, perhaps by asking if there is anything else, move into position three.

STEP 3

Again, break state from position two by going into neutral and thinking about something unrelated, where you are going on holiday, or what you are doing tonight. Now stand back from both previous positions and look at them both as if from a removed point of view. You are attempting to be a judge and adviser to yourself, the fly on the wall, an outside observer. You are not you. Advise you from this removed position and answer these questions:

1. Look at both persons one and two. What can you see that they cannot see? What advice would you offer to person one?

2. What could person one do differently to improve the situation?

3. Are there other suggestions that you can make to person one?

4. Can you find one more thing to suggest to person one?

The effect of these questions and answers is to bring out new possibilities that may not have been thought of before. These insights are discovered having experienced the various alternative positions. Inevitably, therefore, there will be new learning and new ideas. When you are ready, move back to your original position one and become you.

STEP 4

Test by going back to position one (this stage is often referred to as 'reintegration'):

1. Have you now experienced new ideas and perspectives?
2. How differently do you feel about the situation now?
3. What practical steps might you take to move the situation forward?
4. When will you take these steps?

Allow plenty of time for this new information and for emerging feelings towards the situation to come through into your system and your awareness. When you are ready, apply your new awareness.

STEP 5

1. Imagine putting into practice the new behaviours, feelings and actions concerning the issue with which you are dealing.
2. How do you feel now about facing a similar situation in the future?
3. Are you ready to begin taking a new approach to your problem?
4. Is there anything else you need to do? If so do it.

REVIEW

Ask these questions of yourself:

- What is your experience of using this technique of perceptual positioning?
- Have you gained a new perspective, a reframe?
- What has this opportunity to step back given you?
- How practical is it to use this technique in your working life?
- Can you think of other possible uses for this technique, such as preparing for a difficult meeting?

Things to notice when using perceptual positioning

As you moved between the three circles, you might have been aware of being more comfortable in one of them. You might also have noticed being more uncomfortable in one of them. This is a common experience. Depending on our own experience in dealing with the situation, our life patterns, or our roles at work, it could well be that you prefer circle one rather than looking back at yourself from circle two. Equally, you might have found circle two very comfortable and found circle three difficult to stand in.

The model suggests that we should seek to become equally skilled in operating within each sphere at any specific time. The more often the technique is used, the more skilled we become in each circle.

Deepening our understanding: the value of each circle

Position 1

It is essential in dealing with any difficult situation that we are clear about the outcome that we want. We need to have a clear picture of how we would like to sort out the issue in an ideal world. In doing this, we have to identify our positive intentions in dealing with the issue, and towards any other people who are involved. This helps us to clarify our position. It is surprising how many of us are not clear when we are in a compromised situation. We often realise what we don't want rather than being clear about what we actually do want. Children are very clear about what they want in any particular situation, and are often very assertive in telling us what that is! Remember also that you get what you focus on, so focus on what you want.

As we grow up, we are often encouraged not to identify what we want. We are told that if we do we are being selfish and not putting other people first. Can you remember how many times you were told during your own schooling, and throughout childhood, to put other people's needs ahead of your own? However, as this model shows us, if we are unable to identify honestly our needs (to whatever extent), we will be unable to accept another person's wishes without feeling some element of frustration and resentment. This is why it is essential to identify how you are feeling in circle one when you are associated into the problem, as it tells you that the situation as it stands now is not bearable or useful to you and needs to be changed.

Position 2

This is in my experience where the most critical learning occurs. We often pride ourselves as health professionals on being empathetic and understanding. However, this second position consistently proves that we can be much more so, and need to look even deeper into the other person's world. The key here is to cut off from being in position one. When I am using this exercise, participants often blur the two positions and, without realising it, move back to being 'themselves' as one while standing in circle two. This discipline of staying as the other person is where learning is made and it is why it is often useful to have someone talk you through the process, someone who can prompt you if you start to talk as 'I' or 'me'. Learning occurs especially in asking two key questions.

Firstly, how do you, as one, appear to them (you, as you stand in two looking back at yourself)? The reaction is not always pleasant. As they look back at the mirror image of themselves, while they are associated into the problem as the other person, people have described their conduct variously as: 'Petty . . . getting in the way . . . unapproachable . . . fussy . . . dictatorial . . . distant'. None of these behaviours are what we would see from position one in ourselves or would be what we intend. This represents huge learning and self-discovery.

Secondly, what are the other person's positive intentions? As you have probably discovered, these can be very hard to identify. This is the critical moment of learning and is further explored in the key points below. It is worth bearing in mind that anyone's actions and behaviours will be driven by a positive intention from their perspective. Can we, from our perspective, find it, identify with it and allow it into our system to change or modify our view? Perceptual positioning enables us to do this, by thinking things through from their perspective.

Position 3

This is the stepping back position. Many people find this difficult because it is intended to act as a colder, more removed position from which it is possible to reflect rationally and logically. People think it is an uncaring position, because it asks us to remain unassociated. However, one of the consistent findings in working with this technique in practice is that participants are so involved in their issue or problem that they fail to use this position at all, unless prompted to do so.

It is essential therefore that we allow ourselves time to stand or sit in this position. Do not rush things, and do not go for the quick fix. Be aware that you might think that you have come up with, and tried, all of these ideas before, and they haven't worked. This might well be the case, but it is likely that, with your new learning from positions one and two, those old approaches will now work differently, and you will be surprised just how easily you can be successful in resolving the issue. The circumstances have changed due to your use of perceptual positioning, revealing how it is possible to find brand new approaches to dealing with any situation if we allow ourselves the time and we use tried-and-tested techniques.

Again it is important to remain in the correct position here, if you slip back into position one or two it can be useful to physically step backwards, introducing more physical distance, or consider standing on a chair to 'look down on' the situation, literally changing the perspective again, taking care not to put yourself in danger by ensuring the chair is stable and strong enough to hold your weight.

The rewards of using perceptual positioning

The benefits of using this technique of perceptual positioning, and the huge improvements it can create in your state of mind and in your overall efficiency at work, should not be underestimated. It can allow you to be a key player in the resolution of damaging conflicts whether you are directly involved or whether you are helping others. It can create a much more comfortable and productive rapport between yourself and your colleagues, especially those with whom you perhaps do not share an immediate affinity, someone who does something a different way or someone from a different professional discipline. It can also permanently relieve that corrosive, unsettling sense that people are not pulling in the same direction, and that the effectiveness of the whole work project is being compromised by latent, unspoken conflicts of interest and approach.

Just think how much happier you would be in your employment if you could be instrumental in initiating some of these improvements! We would all like to be free of the feeling of dread and demoralisation at going in for a day's work that we know will inevitably contain the subdued threat of conflict or confrontation. By using the step-by-step techniques outlined above, you will feel empowered to forestall those imminent conflicts before they can take root and can begin to damage the effective operation of employees and organisations alike.

So, by becoming a skilful and habitual user of perceptual positioning, you can stifle at origin the sources of so much worry and stress. This is no small matter. Just think how many employees in all sorts of professions crave an antidote to the small, nagging work problems that can accumulate, and can become such a burdensome obstacle to a satisfying sense of fulfilment and which can restrict progression and effective team working. Perceptual positioning offers us a vital reassurance that such obstacles are surmountable with patience and effort and a desire to make life even easier.

The key stages of the journey

You will appreciate that perceptual positioning offers significant rewards, but it also requires effort, time, commitment and understanding. It is therefore worth reviewing the demands, and the benefits of each individual step in order to become as familiar and comfortable as possible with the overall process. Just reflect again on the stages of the journey through the sequence of perceptual positions.

Position 1 This stage involves being clear about how the problem I am confronting is truthfully affecting me emotionally. It involves finding appropriate language to describe my feelings and reactions. It also involves me identifying my positive intentions in the situation.

Position 2 This part of the process involves seeking the positive intentions behind the other person's actions and behaviours. Sometimes people are unable to answer this question, they cannot find any, or simply don't believe that the other person, whose actions have had such a negative effect, are being anything other than awkward, obstructive and bloody-minded. However, everyone's actions and behaviours, no matter how bizarre from where we stand, will have positive intentions from where they stand. The key is for us to uncover them for ourselves, and if we can do this, the discoveries and rewards can be immense. Suddenly we can hear ourselves describing that they too feel isolated, angry, confused, often the mirror image of our own responses. It can be a truly revealing moment when we discover this. Peter's story (p. 122) describes just such a moment of illumination.

Position 3 This stage involves finding new ideas, and revisiting ideas that have already been tried, but now adding a fresh or refreshed perspective. In position three we can suggest anything that might make the difference and offer a solution. These ideas might appear impractical when suggested from position three, but do not edit here. The significance is that you are suggesting ideas for yourself. You now own them, and can test them to see if they work. Simply suggest and discover. Their relevance will be applied and tested in position one when we move back to reintegration. It is surprising how many people uncover the same learning in position three. They say things like:

'I need to meet with them and talk more often . . .'

'I need to step back and give them more room . . .'

'I need to leave it alone . . . remove myself . . . it isn't doing me any good . . .'

This learning isn't hugely scientific or complicated from the outside, looking in. However, it can be immense in relative terms for the individuals concerned, as it moves them on so decisively from the stagnant positions, and the feeling that all options are exhausted, with which they have often struggled for long periods of time.

The following case study vividly illustrates the sort of rapid and fundamental transformations in working relationships that can be brought about by the use of this technique. Here is Jennifer's story.

Jennifer's Story

I was working in my first post in healthcare, as a newly qualified graduate, and my role involved implementing a range of statutory changes within a specific department. It was a fairly high-profile and demanding position, but I had achieved a good degree, and the feedback I was receiving from professionals whom I respected indicated that I was performing the role to a good standard.

However, from the outset I felt hostility from my manager, with whom I was supposed to be coordinating the changes. She had been in her post for over 30 years, and was only a few years from retirement. There were inevitable differences in our backgrounds and approach. A degree was not a requirement when she began work in healthcare, and she was accustomed to the working practices that it was now my job to review. In addition to this, my physical stature is far from imposing, and at the time I looked considerably younger, and more naïve, than my years.

The manager refused point blank to implement many of the changes I suggested, and at times would even refuse to sit down with me to discuss options. Her manner was cold and confrontational, she referred to me in terms that I found demeaning, and I felt that her way of running the department was becoming increasingly autocratic and inflexible. Dislike and resentment seemed to dictate her attitude towards me. The situation had become almost intolerable, and had reached a point where I was ready to resign.

One day, I was sitting in a coffee shop with a member of the support staff, describing my frustration at the way things were going. Having listened to my problems, she suggested a short exercise that might help. She asked me to sit at a different chair at the table, and imagine as fully as possible what it must be like to be my manager. She then asked me to look across at where I had been sitting, and try to experience what my manager's feelings towards me must be. 'Dislike' and 'resentment' came to me immediately. But then, I suddenly said 'scared', and remarkably I started to cry. As my manager, I felt an overwhelming sense of threat, fear and vulnerability. From the point of view of the manager, as I looked at 'myself' across the table, I thought, 'She's trying to get me out of my job.' I saw that anxiety and insecurity were at the source of my manager's behaviour.

My colleague then directed me to a third chair – the coffee shop was fairly empty – and asked me to say what advice I would offer to the person sitting in the first chair to make the situation better. I said that she should ask her manager to come on board with her in what she was aiming to do, and ask for help with her task. She should request that the manager work with her on the project, and she should enquire whether it would be possible to shadow her for a day in order to build up her understanding of the demands of the manager's role.

I returned to work with a new and refreshed sense of purpose. I put into practice all of the strategies suggested by the 'third party', and our relationship improved immeasurably. Although I have now moved on from my work in that department, the long-term shift in my relationship with my manager brought about a good year of constructive and cooperative work together.

It is worth just reviewing the benefits of using perceptual positioning in this way.

- First, it places responsibility on us to look 'at cause' rather than be 'in effect' (see Chapter 2). Very often we seek to blame others, think that we have exhausted all options and energy, and we become stuck by giving up on them. The perceptual positioning process gives us options, and asks us to look at ourselves in a new light.

- Second, it emphasises gains for each party involved. I will only be able to reintegrate ideas from position three back into one if they offer me and the other party a 'win'. Otherwise, it will fail as a suggested way forward. So my thinking in position three has to be practical, realistic and ecological, appropriate and in the best interests of all parties involved.

- Third, it is a flexible tool, adaptable over time and within a wide range of different situations. If I try a solution that emerges from the 'three circle' process, and it either works for a short time or not at all, then I can reuse it to revisit the situation again at a later date, and perhaps find a more lasting resolution to the problem. I can also use the tool in other situations once I am familiar with it.

- Fourth, it reduces stress caused by being stuck. We fool ourselves that we are 'just dealing with this kind of situation, because that is the way it is . . .' Underneath this passive acceptance, we can be causing ourselves real damage by living in effect. It need not be this way, as the technique demonstrates.

- Fifth, it is adaptable for both my own coaching of me, and for when others are coaching me, or I am coaching them. I have known teams of people within the same organisation using this and offering to walk each other round the three circles (in the privacy of a closed space!). It can help bring colleagues together, and become closer and more effective in their jobs. Equally, I can talk or walk myself through the three positions and get a changed perspective for myself, surprisingly quickly.

- Sixth, it is content free. If I am working with someone else either as a coach or facilitator, then I need know nothing of the issue that they are dealing with.

It might even be about me, although I wouldn't advise this! The attraction of being content free is that as the coach I can remain at a distance, not falling into the trap of becoming an adviser or mentor or confidant. The suggestions will be much more powerful coming from the person involved since they know what they need to do to gain an effective resolution. Instead, I am free to concentrate on the process and on observing my colleague as they move around the three circles. Am I asking the questions at the correct time? Am I giving them enough time to reflect? Do I need to ask the question again? Are they remaining in the correct position at each stage? By reflecting on these elements of my own role, I can oversee the process and act as a facilitator.

Important footnote

I would just like to offer a word of caution. When working with another person, or in asking another person to work with you, please do not use this technique to explore traumatic situations. These situations, such as loss or injury, can often unlock deeply held emotions, which need to be cleared with a qualified coach before using this technique. The power of these emotions, especially when entering position two, can become overwhelming. The tool is therefore inappropriate in these circumstances, as it will offer little progress towards any form of resolution.

It will be useful to consolidate the ideas contained in this chapter by considering a final case study. Read through Peter's account of using perceptual positioning in conflict resolution, and then reflect on any parallels with your own day-to-day experiences at work.

Peter's Story

Peter managed three teams within his responsibilities. They all had similar functions, and were spread over a wide region. They were all staffed the same way, and had the same level of autonomy. Two of the teams responded well to Peter's way of managing them. He managed them at arm's length, but was clear about how they should report to him, and by what timetable they should respond each month. The third team was managed in exactly the same way, and yet was consistently late with their monthly returns, or never sent them at all. They failed to respond to email requests, and even after being visited failed to make the changes Peter asked them to make. Peter had given up on this team, was very unhappy about it and believed that their way of doing things was 'personal' and amounted to an attack on his authority.

In walking through the three circles, Peter found it almost impossible to find any positive intentions behind their actions. 'There aren't any,' he said, over and over again. Peter was trapped in circle one feeling personally affronted, and moved to circle three without spending long enough in circle two. I asked Peter to challenge himself and to find a positive intention behind their apparent lack of cooperation in failing to respond to his requests. When I asked him to talk me through his responses whilst standing in circle two, the conversation went like this.

Q: What do these people feel like who make up this team?
P (after pausing): They just don't like the way I manage them. They don't like me.

Q: Can you find a positive intention behind this not liking you?
P: They want to avoid me.

Q: And what is the positive intention behind avoiding you?
P: Not having to fill in their returns and carry out their responsibilities.

Q: And what is their positive intention in doing this?
P: They don't want to show that they have failed to meet their monthly targets.

Q: And what does this mean about their positive intentions?
P (after pausing again): That they are hiding.

Q: And this means what?
P: That they are afraid.

Q: And what is the positive intention behind this fear?
P: (after another pause, this one long): That they might lose their jobs if they tell me what is really happening.

Q: And what is the positive intention here?
P (after a shorter pause): They want to protect themselves and their team . . .

Here I witnessed a huge physiological shift in Peter's tone, body language and facial expression. He almost smiled, and started to move from one foot to another, as if he was lighter on his feet.

Q: And knowing this, how might you appear to them in the way you have handled the situation?
P (after a pause): I might look pushy, efficient . . . a bit of a threat?

Q: OK – would you now like to leave this circle and move to position three?
P: Yes.

Understanding this fear of job losses and the possible break-up of their team, (their map), Peter was able to move to position three and suggest new ways that he could meet with them, ask for the information, and reassure them directly on the issue of job losses.

On re-entering position one, he felt more relaxed. He could see a way of starting to sort out the problem, and his anger had subsided.

However, on one thing he was very clear. We agreed it did not excuse the way that they had handled the situation by simply ignoring Peter's requests for information. In Peter's eyes this was still an abdication of responsibility and highly disrespectful to his way of trying to manage them and go about his job. However he now understood their motivation, the cause, and he could move on to find a more constructive path, hopefully for himself and his team.

Summary

Reframing through the skill of perceptual positioning is an immensely productive way of discovering, through reflection, solutions for problems or issues that might have left us with a sense of hopelessness or inertia. Like any other skill, it requires practice, but through regular use it can become integrated into our thinking, and can be gradually refined as a means of dealing with conflict.

As Peter's case study shows, the technique encourages us to look at the cause of a situation instead of persevering 'in effect'. It challenges us to reconsider how we see other people, and ourselves. It helps us to unlock and broaden our map of the territory. In this sense, it can be revealing, and we may not always like what we see. It is vital to accept the key principle that all actions and behaviours, no matter how misdirected or random or ill thought through, either by us or by other people, have a positive intention. If we allow ourselves to find this positive intention and to accept it, any situation will begin to change, and will represent itself differently in our minds, for the better.

It is essential to reiterate a crucial point. As Peter's story demonstrates, the skill of perceptual positioning does not ask us to accept and tolerate another person's conduct or actions. Peter still believed the team's way of handling the original problem was badly misdirected. However, he did not let that get in the way of resolving the stand-off, and discovering a way forward.

Having journeyed through the three positions, discovered positive intentions, seen our own approach in a new light, and uncovered new ways forward in dealing with the issue, it does not mean that I have to accept that the other person is correct or justified in their views and the way that they have dealt with the situation. On the contrary, it might well show me that my approach has been equally justified and valid, and that the best thing I can do is to keep to my course of action. I may well change how I implement my decisions; for example I might intervene less or more depending on the situation. However, my conviction remains the same; and having understood the range of people's feelings and motives more fully, I am no longer allowing myself to doubt, berate and stress myself as I had been doing before I began the search for a positive resolution. I now truly have a fresh perspective.

The technique of perceptual positioning of course has deeper resonance beyond the resolution of workplace conflicts, valuable though this is. To return to the issues introduced at the opening of the chapter, Augustus Casely-Hayford writes of:

> ' . . . the need to find a new infrastructure, an integrated mechanism for thinking about how demographic changes alter the way metropolitan Britons engage with the world around them.'

He also emphasises that 'generating formalised ways to accommodate "other" people and then not resourcing or embracing the complexity of that responsibility can actually exacerbate the problem'. Perceptual positioning can offer an invaluable resource in the journey towards embracing the new realities surrounding us, both in the workplace and in the much broader world beyond.

Reference

Grinder, J., De Lozier, J. (1996) *Turtles all the Way Down: Prerequisites to personal genius*. Portland, Oregon, Metamorphous Press.

Goal setting

Jim Lister

7

Is there a risk that you restrict your achievements by not setting high enough goals?

By now you will have been asking yourself lots of questions about who you are, what you believe, how you work and how you manage difficult situations. You may also have begun to consider what it is you want more of in your professional and personal life. But how many times have you sat down and seriously considered your purpose for living? Our 'purpose for living' is a huge question, one that we often reflect on briefly, but then prefer to put to one side. After all, there is no easy answer, and the question requires us to look long and hard at ourselves. And self-scrutiny is not always the most comfortable of activities, unless, that is, we are well prepared, and understand that there is a system with which to elicit the answers we desire. This chapter will provide techniques that will help you to ask the big, enduring questions about your life's objectives and destiny. The answers you will uncover can offer immeasurable, fundamental benefits for your career and for your wider life.

Initially, it is also worth asking whether you already set yourself goals, perhaps for the longer, medium and short term. In all likelihood, the answer to this question is 'Yes', though you probably do it subconsciously, without really thinking it through. After all, goals are how we move ourselves forward, how we make mundane decisions such as getting up in the morning, dressing for the day, eating, working, relaxing and sleeping. We rarely consider these activities to be 'goals' as such, simply an essential way in which we conduct our lives and progress through the days, but they do represent 'goal setting' of a basic, almost instinctive kind.

The benefits of refining and heightening these innate skills can be truly profound. There is nothing arrogant or self-absorbed about defining a firm set of goals and committing yourself to achieving them. However, as a society we seem to be remarkably diffident about the process. As Sue Knight (2002, p. 263) observes, statistics indicate that 'only six percent of the population thinks strategically, and this includes the ability to set and hold compelling goals'. If you are to reap the benefits of becoming skilled at goal setting, an essential first step must be to dispel the inner dialogue whispering that you are unworthy of the rewards that come with aspiring to ambitious targets. Confining yourself to low aspirations is not an admirable sign of modesty or self-effacement. As Joseph O'Connor (2001, p. 19) pithily observes, 'Modesty means not bragging about what you can do.' You need to be determined from the outset to bracket yourself with those people whose success in life is based on skilled goal setting.

Goal setting in healthcare

The concept of goal setting applies to healthcare workers in ways that differ significantly from other professionals. At the source of a healthcare worker's motivation must be concern for the comfort and well-being of others, and minimising the suffering of patients will inevitably comprise the fundamental inspiration and purpose of the vast majority of people when they enter the profession. To talk of these motives in terms of goals and targets might seem cold, even robotic. Many people in healthcare make their initial choice to enter the profession through a sense of vocation, often motivated by sensitive personal experiences that make them at once vulnerable, and also determined to make healthcare their calling. It would surely be a rare healthcare worker who would not cite as a key motivation the desire to make a difference to the lives of other people, to gain satisfaction in their careers and lives through helping to relieve the distress of people who are suffering with illness and disease.

These considerations make it all the harder for healthcare professionals to separate personal goals and an overall life purpose, from professional targets. Whilst it might be a sweeping generalisation, business people and sales people, shopkeepers and stockbrokers, do not need to factor into the calculation of their goals the extent to which they are meeting the needs of vulnerable people. In fact, it may well impede the achievement of their targets were they to get sidetracked in this way. Healthcare workers, however, must inevitably measure themselves by the extent to which they have contributed to their patients' comfort and recovery from illness. This obviously makes goal setting a more subtle and delicate process for a healthcare worker than it would be for a sales person whose targets will be based solely on the number of items shifted, or the amount of revenue generated.

However, it might also be a distortion to over-exaggerate the vocational factors behind a healthcare worker's choice of career. People choose the profession for a wide range of reasons; we feel we have the particular talents to succeed and gain promotion through the ranks, we are attracted by the challenge, the lifestyle, the hours, the camaraderie, or we like the security of working for a large, perhaps publicly funded organisation. The balance between altruistic and self-serving motives is in all likelihood very subtle and difficult to quantify, and it is probably in a continual state of flux.

Establishing your life purpose, your goals and your targets, will take all of these factors into consideration. A goal such as 'to make as big a difference to as many patients' lives as possible' might, while being an admirable and authentic goal, be a little too vague to be measurable and truly achievable. On the other hand, 'to cure at least 65% of my patients, rising to 70% next year' might be just as unfeasible, not to say crass. If we are to align our goals with our deeper beliefs and values, they must contain an element of the ideals and altruistic motives that inspired us to become a healthcare professional in the first place. However, they must also be closely aligned with the kind of tangible professional achievements that are integrated into the personal goal setting process that is integral to all jobs in the modern world. Single-minded personal ambition is nothing to be ashamed of here; after all, if healthcare professionals are performing efficiently as measured by externally established standards, patient care must, as a natural consequence, improve accordingly.

This chapter will seek to highlight and cultivate the talents we all possess in the area of target setting, in defining our goals and working towards the outcomes we desire. Being clear about desired outcomes can make us stronger and more confident, better equipped to believe in ourselves so that we feel able to manage our working lives even more successfully. In addition, clear and decisive goal setting enables us to handle professional change in a way that controls and neutralises the accompanying threat of stress and anxiety. Earlier we urged you to start living your dream. Goal setting gives you a tool to make that reality.

Dreaming is a great start. In order to realise your dream you need structure, you need plans and a clear deadline. Then you need to take the first step. Without that it remains just a pleasant dream.

Life purpose and vision

Your vision represents the 'big picture' of your life. It can, if you wish, be narrowed down to focus on the more specific area of your working life, and this chapter will pose numerous questions for you to consider. Make your own choice now, before you go on: are you going to answer these questions from your overall life perspective, or from the perspective of your professional life? Certainly the two are inextricably linked, and starting with your 'working life' vision will present solutions relevant to your wider life, so it might be useful to begin here. You can always return to do your overall life perspective at a later date.

The starting point is the question of fulfilment. What is it that serves as your vision, or purpose, and drives you to be a healthcare professional? My guess is that you may have responded with a tentative, 'Never really thought about it before.' Most of us, after all, have never considered the question of our broader 'purpose' or direction, choosing to carry on our lives without ever establishing our vision. So what is to be gained by coming up with an answer? The undeniable truth is that we can be more motivated when our values, beliefs, actions and overarching sense of identity are all in line, all congruent, unified and fulfilled. We become happier, more motivated and more productive.

Before exploring how to establish your vision, consider your working life at the moment. How content and fulfilled are you? What does your Wheel of Life look like? (Chapter 4.) Do you experience a split between what you want to do and what you actually do? (See Chapter 9.) How useful and manageable is that split? Is it long-term, or more recently emerging? Wouldn't it be great actually to do what you really want to do? Does this sound so unrealistic? It doesn't have to be, and taking action along the lines suggested in this chapter will inevitably help you to recognise that desire and reality are in fact compatible. It might sound like a cliché, but if we wish, we can live our dreams, rather than pretending not to have any in case they are not fulfilled. By accepting this idea, you will be able to move on from simple, day-to-day living and target setting, gradually embracing a more purposeful, compelling and dynamic existence. Just take a few moments to consider what it would feel like if you had a clear sense of purpose in your life and work, and you were working in such a way that you knew you were moving towards meeting that. Just how good does that feel?

Creating your life purpose

Before we look any further, consider this short exercise. It will help to bring into sharper focus any intuitions about your life's goals that might exist at a subconscious level.

Exercise 7.1
Finding My Life Purpose

Sit quietly, somewhere you can think properly, where you can really concentrate on yourself. Write a short statement that encapsulates your feelings about your life purpose, your vision. It should summarise how you would like your working life to be and how you will achieve a sense of fulfilment as a healthcare professional. Jamie Smart (www.Saladltd.co.uk) poses what he calls the 'miracle question':

'If there was a miracle tonight, and when you woke up tomorrow, everything [in this area of your life/work/business] was exactly as you'd like it to be, how would you know a miracle had occurred? What would you see, hear, feel and believe that would let you know it had happened?'

When you have done this, ask yourself, 'Is this all I would like it to be?' If you feel the answer is 'no' ask yourself: 'Is there something else that I can add to make it even more powerful, so that I feel even more fulfilled?' This is not an intellectual process. It is instead something that should emerge from a deeper place within you. Give yourself time to think about it, listen to your inner voice and any prompts it gives you. Have the courage to ask your subconscious mind to reveal your vision to you. You will be surprised at just how easily your subconscious mind will respond when you ask it a direct question. Write down whatever emerges.

Just take a moment to read back what you have written. Does it make you excited? Can you see what it would look like, hear what it would sound like and feel what it would feel like? Even now are new ideas coming into your head to build on and put detail around that vision? If it doesn't make you feel a bit insecure and a bit nervous, you have not arrived at your vision. It should feel big, it should feel slightly beyond your reach at this stage and it should make you want to run out to meet it and live it. Have you found your vision yet?

The importance of consulting your subconscious

Our minds are comprised of two functions, the conscious and the subconscious. Although it is inevitably beyond the scope of the current book to become immersed in detailed examinations of these two functions, brief definitions of what we mean when applying the labels will obviously be helpful here. Our conscious, rational thought process keeps us going throughout our daily lives. Joseph O'Connor (2001, p. 281) succinctly defines the 'conscious' as 'anything in present-moment awareness'. It is the state in which we are aware of controlling our thought patterns, and it makes us practical and logical. It allows us to store tasks and presents them so that we can complete them.

Underneath this, however, lies the deeper stratum of the mind, the unknown, and we refer to this source of hidden potential as our subconscious. This is where we store our memories and our dreams, our untapped creativity, and it can act as an enormous resource if we can find conscious ways in which to explore and release the energies within. Sue Knight (2002, p. 274) explains the crucial role played by the subconscious in the process of goal setting: 'your unconscious mind does not differentiate between what is imagined and what is real. The more vividly you imagine yourself achieving what you want, the more your unconscious mind believes it already has it and will programme you to act as if you do.' Embedding your goals and aspirations, indeed your life's vision, deep within your subconscious is far from being some kind of unfocused, fanciful superstition. In the words of W.B. Yeats (1990), 'In dreams begins responsibility'.

A further metaphor will help to compound your appreciation of the importance of recruiting the vast untapped reserves of creativity and energy in your subconscious. In his book *The Power of Your Sub-Conscious Mind*, Joseph Murphy (1988, p. 6) describes the subconscious as a 'bed of rich soil that will help all kinds of seeds to sprout and flourish. Plant wonderful seeds of thought in the garden of your mind and you will reap a glorious harvest'. And it is remarkable just how often people find that fate seems to work in their favour when they sincerely commit themselves to honest, worthwhile goals, goals which are congruent with their values and beliefs.

Rather than neglecting the subconscious, or treating it with suspicion, we need to recognise it as an astonishingly fertile reservoir for ideas, plans and initiatives. We need to start using the whole of our minds and not limit our potential by ignoring that our sub-conscious exists.

So, if you have not yet established your vision revisit Exercise 7.1 and switch off your conscious mind and listen to that inner voice which so wants to help you to achieve all that you were created to achieve.

Exercise 7.2
Taking Charge of My Thought Processes

So, how do we go about planting these seeds of thought in the fertile ground of the subconscious? Quite simply by requesting, suggesting and consulting through taking charge of our thought processes. Here is a suggested sequence of exercises:

In a quiet space tell your mind and body to relax. Do whatever you need to do to relax fully. Sit comfortably, remove any likely disturbances and focus fully on you.

Relax the muscles round your eyes and then across your face.

Relax your tongue, let it fall from the roof of your mouth.

Listen to and feel your own breathing for five minutes and really be aware of it.

Breathe out any tension and any negative emotions which might prevent you from hearing your inner voice.

Focus your attention on seeking your purpose in life by asking yourself to provide the answer. Your unconscious mind responds well to commands.

Allow answers to appear. Listen to your inner voice.

Focus on how you wish to feel if you had such a purpose available to you *now*.

Enjoy playing with that sensation and stay with it for a further five minutes.

See it, hear it, feel it. Make the picture as big and bright as you can.

Bring yourself back into the conscious world and as you go about your daily tasks, listen inside to whether the answers which emerge fit your true life purpose.

Repeat as often as you wish – no charge, except on your time!

You are trying to connect with what really motivates you, or what has historically motivated you. If you could do anything, what would it be? Look again at your work values and consider how they can be fulfilled (Chapter 5). If you think back to when you were a child, you will remember that you were probably more in touch with your intuitions and your dreams. Can you imagine how great it would be to be able to reconnect with them?

Just take a moment to consider how this process of inner reflection has helped to reinforce your life purpose. Do you have a clear idea of where you want to get to and how you want to be? What new stimuli did the process uncover which you can use to motivate the current you towards this new future you?

Of course, we have to understand the need to seek out realistic possibilities that provide us with evidence that our vision or dream is achievable. This motivates us even more. It is striking this balance between the bigger dreams and the achievable outcomes that is the key to finding our life purpose. This in turn will drive us into action via goal setting.

The implications of finding a renewed life purpose

It is important to reflect on the depth and significance of what is being asked here in considering this vision. It could be that you are about to change direction from a path that you have been on for many years, or make significant changes along the same path. This will have implications for you and for many other people around you. To whatever extent, you might be about to upset the status quo which has formed the basis for your life. You are potentially entering new territory. It is therefore essential to consult others in drawing together your vision statement, especially family, friends and colleagues. Consider how your new or re-emphasised vision might affect them, and ask for their thoughts. Ask them for their support in your new direction, get them involved and consider how you will continue to relate to them. This is a vital part of setting the scene for your new mission and making it happen.

And how do we know after all this that we have succeeded in finding our purpose? By sensing it, by feeling positive each morning as we get up to go to work. We will begin to approach our lives with an intensity and passion which is truly fulfilling.

To illustrate the implications of defining a new vision or a set of goals, Joanne recalls an experience in which her determination to follow a specific career option resulted in wider repercussions for her home life.

Joanne's Story

I was already employed in a fairly demanding post as a healthcare lecturer, when an opportunity arose to contribute to the work of a multi-disciplinary team implementing some groundbreaking initiatives with children's bereavement groups. I felt that it was interesting and vital work, which I knew I would find exacting but stimulating. The team was full of energy and expertise, exploring practical ways of dealing with child bereavement, and I quickly found that it was taking up a lot of time on top of my primary work as a lecturer. However, it was a direction I wished to go in, and I felt that I was coping with both roles without it affecting my home life.

I had two fairly young children at the time, and one day they suddenly asked me if they could come along to the bereavement group, as they wanted to take part in all the fun things they'd seen me preparing at home. It came as a bit of a shock to realise that they saw this as the only way they could spend any prolonged time with their mother. In spite of my professional commitments, I felt that I had been managing to supply their needs. The discovery that this had not been the case required me to reassess things and make adjustments to the balance between my work and my wider life. I have made sure to stay vigilant about the balance between professional goals and my broader life commitments since this experience.

This story illustrates the importance of checking out how changes you make affect others.

Joanne also offers some interesting observations on the implications of utilising NLP in a healthcare context and how this has helped her rediscover a deeper life purpose within her professional practice.

I see the integration of NLP into every aspect of my professional practice as a primary vision in itself. I now use the NLP techniques that I have built up over the years absolutely instinctively in all my work, and I feel strongly that this has brought great benefits. Colleagues do comment directly to me that I seem to be able to cope with stressful and difficult situations in a comparatively calm and unruffled way. I have to remind them that this does not simply happen, but requires considerable preparation, care and thought just beneath the surface!

The rewards of using NLP in terms of increased competence and improved professional performance are substantial, but they don't come without a price. Time, commitment, forethought are all needed in abundance, and you have to guard against becoming too introverted or self-analytical. There is a risk of becoming isolated because of the specific choices you make, and there is no point disguising the fact that some colleagues are doubtful, even openly scep-tical, about the whole counselling process. The issue of ecology becomes very important here. I regularly assess the implications of my commitment to NLP for the wider picture of my life. For example, I have to make choices about the relationships I wish to retain in the light of people's responses to the directions in which NLP takes me. Whilst there is undoubtedly a price to pay, for me the benefits greatly outweigh the sacrifices, and I am content with the balance I have found. I now know what I want to achieve in life, I know what I can contribute.

Goal setting

So far, we have suggested that you look at the deeper purpose of your working life and construct a meaningful, relevant and inspiring vision statement. We have recommended that you reflect inwards, by taking time to refer to your sub-conscious to define what it is you really want. By following this process you will have identified your life's great desires, as well as some of your deepest values. It is well worth referring back to Chapter 5 on Values to ensure that you have aligned your vision statement with your deep-rooted beliefs and values. Most importantly, as Steve Andreas and Charles Faulkener emphasise in their book *NLP: The New*

Technology of Achievement (1994, p. 105), 'Make it fit into the essential paradox of a mission: something you can never finish, but that you can do every day.'

If this vision statement becomes firmly established at the forefront of your thoughts, and is true to you and your needs, then inevitably you will be motivated into action. Equally, it will help prepare you for whatever you encounter on the journey towards fulfilling your purpose, the changes you will be required to make, the stresses, the unexpected twists and turns. These challenges will be easier to face once you have defined a firm sense of purpose that is driving you into the future.

It is suggested that you discover your vision statement before carrying on with this chapter. It will serve as a vital prelude to the deeper understanding of goal setting that you are now about to explore.

Choosing your goals

Having established or reconfirmed your life purpose, how do you intend to go about living it and embodying it in your life so that you enact it successfully and effectively? After all, people will not judge you simply on the quality of your vision. You will of course be judged on your actions and behaviour, the things that people see you doing, as you set about enacting your mission and achieving success. As suggested already, we can focus or frame this 'enacting' by setting out what it is we wish to achieve through the clear establishment of goals.

Quite simply, goals are our intentions, and they should be clearly stated, carefully thought through, and preferably written down for reinforcement. A clear deadline and timetable will enable you to measure whether or not your goals have been attained. And as we have already discovered, they are most likely to be successfully achieved if they are driven by and linked inextricably with an identified life purpose.

Choice is at the heart of effective goal setting. Twenty-first-century society offers us potentially unlimited choice, and in order to cope with this we constantly have to narrow down our options by hopefully making the choices that will satisfy us. If our vision is our fullest potential, our eventual destination, then our specific goals can become the route by which we get there. They allow us to check that we have arrived, or at least are on track.

Therefore goals can represent a present-day view of what we intend to achieve in the future as an essential component of our overall vision. The more that we think about our goals, see them in our mind's eye, hear them, and feel the effects of what it might be like to achieve them, the more success we will encounter in our endeavours. This is because goal setting allows us to choose effective action in order to fulfil our wishes. Goals motivate the conscious and the subconscious mind by providing direction. So, how do we become effective at setting and achieving goals?

The practice – specifying and recording your goals

There are three 'levels' at which goals can be set:

- Long term – designed to give overall shape and direction to your life;
- Medium term – lying underneath your long-term goals and supporting them;
- Short term – supporting your medium-term goals and shaping your day-to-day life.

In the past you may have written shorter-term goals which have not been achieved. Did you have a goal beyond the goal? It is important that you know what the goal will achieve for you in order to gain the motivation required to achieve it and go beyond it. Whenever you set a goal ask yourself, 'What will that do for me?' to ensure that you have a goal beyond the goal.

You may in the past also have set a longer-term goal and then lost track of it over time. This may have been due to a lack of short- or medium-term goals which work as steps along the way. The use of all three levels of goal setting helps to avoid some of these common problems within goal setting which you might have experienced in the past. By setting goals at all levels, you will hugely increase your success rates in achieving them.

The final point it is worth raising here about levels of goals is that having set your goals at all three levels, ensure that you identify the first step in the first goal to ensure that you can move very quickly towards achieving your first goal.

Preparing to set goals

It is useful to start with longer-term goals. Using the guidance below (Ten Golden Rules of Goal Setting) write down your long-term goals in a neat and ordered style, and display them, or put them in a place where you will easily be able to access and refer to them, to reinforce your identification with and commitment to them. Having listed them, can you prioritise them?

Having done this for long-term goals, now break each goal down into medium-term goals, and prioritise these.

Now do the same for the medium-term goals, breaking these down into shorter-term goals and again prioritise them in turn. You will have developed a pyramid of goals, all driven by your vision statement or life purpose.

Before we look at a more specific process for setting goals, bringing more firmly into focus the ideas you have already generated, here are a number of criteria to bear in mind as good practice:

Ten golden rules of goal setting

1. Always state your goals in the positive. State what you want rather than what you do not want. This gives greater focus and prevents even part of your mind thinking over what might not happen. Don't give yourself permission to dwell on any negatives!

2. Pursue the goals that you believe in and want. It is often tempting to hear other people's suggestions and take them as your own, especially if they are suggested by your boss or by a colleague you admire. You will only achieve goals that are relevant and meaningful to you, goals that you really want to reach.

3. Set out a practical and realistic timetable with deadlines you can meet. This acts as a powerful motivator. Again, write down your deadlines. Establish the first step towards your goal.

4. List the benefits of achieving your goals, in the longer, medium and short term. Consider your goal beyond your goal: what obtaining your goal will do for you. This discipline will act as a powerful stimulus to staying committed to your goals. These benefits can be wide ranging and long term. They might well affect other people as well as yourself. It is equally useful to detail what you will leave behind or avoid by achieving your goals.

5. Ensure that the ability to achieve your goals lies within your own power as far as possible. For some goals you might need to enlist the help of others. Ask yourself honestly whether you can rely on those people. What proportion in the achievement of your goals are you entrusting to the actions of others? You need to reduce as much as possible the likelihood of being let down by the contribution of other people, or independent external influences.

6. Ensure that all the goals you have identified fit with your values and beliefs. We will look further at this point when we describe the 'ecology' check that we need to make in order to measure the potential impact of our future actions on the status quo. You might identify a goal that seems appropriate now, and yet when you look carefully at the future, you might foresee unintentional fall-out far outweighing the gains originally intended.

7. Write down your goals and display them in a prominent place for your personal reference. Remember though that they are personal to you and should only be shared with those that you trust.

8. Find a mantra or convenient phrase which helps sum up each goal. This helps you remember it and ensures that you keep the goal at the forefront of your mind: remember you get what you focus on, so ensure this is phrased in the positive.

9. Regularly review your goals, annually for the longer term, monthly and weekly, or even daily or hourly, for the medium term to shorter term. You can afford to be flexible! Do not feel that your goals are set in stone. They are susceptible to change and fluctuations, and must be relevant to the conditions and circumstances of your life, which themselves often change. Do not let the goals enslave you, they should help not hinder you in achieving what you want to achieve. If a goal is no longer helpful in achieving your desired outcome, change it or remove it.

10. Challenge yourself and be prepared to move into the learning zone of self-discovery rather than remaining in the familiar comfort or safety zone.

A goal setting process

It is vital to know what you want in order to select your goals, just as it is important to run a check on whether the goals that you have selected will deliver what you want as well as whether or not they are worth having. This ecology or future check is important as we are trying to predict our future by setting goals. What if they don't deliver in the way that we envisaged? The more that we can prepare before setting out on the journey, to ensure that our destination is the one that suits us, the better. Also allow for flexibility, if there is more than one way to achieve a goal do not restrict yourself to only achieving it one way.

It is time now to concentrate on the detailed sequence of activities that will lead to you conclusively identifying and defining your specific goals.

Exercise 7.3
Goal Setting

Work through this sequence carefully and methodically, remembering the importance of recruiting the resources of the subconscious mind. Recall the possibilities and priorities regarding your goals already established in the preceding exercises.

1. Select a Primary Goal.

Choose a longer-term goal that is critical to you fulfilling your life purpose. Listen to your instincts and to your subconscious. Your primary goal should override other, lesser goals, and it should keep coming back to you as the first priority when you are deciding which one to select. It will enable you to fulfil your life purpose more than any other goal. Look ahead between one and three years and think where you wish your career to be at the end of that period. Is it a goal relating to your own personal development, such as being more confident or motivated, or is it aimed at reaching a certain position in your professional practice or employment? Make sure that it is stated in positive terms and is under your control.

Examples might be:

- to be a senior manager in three years
- to be assertive in my work by getting my points across more constructively
- to be a confident presenter and trainer
- to have a new job with a fresh focus for my career within three years

2. Select Medium- and Short-Term Goals.

If you are working to a primary goal that you wish to achieve within a three-year period, start to map out your medium-term goals over each six-month period. These six pieces of the primary goal jigsaw together to make the whole picture. Look at how they fit together and in which order to place them.

Under each of these six medium-term goals, list any number of shorter-term goals to be carried out monthly, weekly and daily. Together this represents your initial action plan that can be reviewed whenever you wish. The more disciplined you can be in writing down your goals, defining them, and looking to see where you have achieved them, the more successful you will become at both measuring and achieving the plan you have established.

3. Provide Evidence that You are Achieving Goals.

The evidence will be based on your actions and achievements. They will also be timetabled and measurable against the deadlines that you set. The more detailed evidence you can provide, the more you will be able to record your progress and either confirm your original action plan, or adjust it. It is crucial to identify the evidence as you set out to achieve your goals.

Evidence of goal achievement can also be established if you vividly imagine where and with whom you want to achieve your goal. This enables you to become more specific and applied and helps you to create a fuller picture of this future event. It becomes more real to you in the present moment, and you will be more motivated to go out and do it because it is already half achieved, at least in your mind's eye.

Many day-to-day tasks will be short-term goals in themselves. It is a surprisingly refreshing exercise to sit down at the end of each day, and tick off and measure the number of tasks that you have achieved. One of the most powerful aspects of skilled goal setting is when you discover that these daily achievements fit within a vision fully in line with an overarching 'life purpose'. Then, an almost magical transformation can occur, and each day, what was an abstract set of identified targets becomes a reality that has been achieved.

4. Conduct an Ecology Check.

This is a vital stage that helps us to avoid the 'whatever it takes' scenario described by Andreas and Faulkener (1994). They show that sometimes in our pursuit of goals we can lose track of the rest of our lives, and seek to deliver them no matter what. The 'whatever it takes' mentality, if it remains unchecked and moves out of line with the rest of our lives, can be inadvertently destructive.

In order to arrest this tendency, we have already considered the bigger picture of our vision, which helps ensure that our goals are a part of our deeper values and the things that we believe in. In addition, we can further check our goals for their 'ecology' within our wider life. Do they fit? Will they create hidden conflicts or tensions either for us, or for other people who are involved, such as family, friends and colleagues? Are there any potentially negative consequences of fulfilling your goals? Can these be turned around into positive outcomes? Does this evidence force you to reconsider and reschedule your goals?

To conduct an ecology check, choose one of your goals. Now imagine yourself looking into the future, having achieved this goal by running through your mind when and where you will be, who will be with you, what is happening and how you will feel. Spend at least five minutes running this programme through your mind, filling in as much detail as possible.

After this, come out of this imaginative state and ask yourself these questions. Did you uncover any negative associations on your journey? How might you avoid these? Are you now able to describe what you will have to let go of or give up in pursuit of the goal, and have you identified the things that you are determined to keep?

What is the impact on other people who are involved? Are there any negative associations with them, and if so, what can you do to prevent them? What else is affected in your life, and what are the costs to you, for example in time and money?

In answering these questions, it should now have become clear that your goal is valid and relevant, and that the benefits far outweigh the costs. If not, it is worth reconsidering your goal.

It would be worth recording your thoughts on a table like the one in Figure 7.1 below.

Specific Goal	Goal Definition	Evidence of Achievement through Actions	Ecology
Primary Long-Term Goal Medium-Term Goals Short-Term Goals			

(A blank version of this form can be found on the website at www.wiley.com/go/ nlphealthcare)

Figure 7.1 Analysis of goals

5. Taking Action

So far, everything has been created solely in your mind: the need, the possibilities, the overall vision, the benefits, the likelihood of success, the evidence, the way that others are involved and the impact on them. This all seems well and good, so now you are ready to move forward and put your ideas into action. It is only through testing and going about achieving your goals in real terms that you will be convinced that you have chosen the correct path.

In Chapter 8 we will look further at how to move forward with your goals by using a specific four-step approach. The starting point for this process is goal setting, so we would urge you to spend time on this here, before moving on.

As we have seen so far, the skill and discipline of goal setting can deliver great success for us in our lives, and can provide a solid foundation on which to start to plan the kind of lives we desire. Goals can quickly begin to move us forward when we become stuck in our professional lives, especially when these goals are closely attached to a grander life purpose that we have signed up to.

Nina's Story

Here is how Nina, when faced with the possibility of redundancy from her job within a healthcare organisation, used the goal setting process to take charge of her future career options (Figure 7.2).

Specific Goal	Goal Definition	Evidence of Achievement through Actions	Ecology
Primary Long-Term Goal	To secure a purposeful, responsible job, in training, strategic planning or operations management, representing promotion from my current post	Being appointed to a job that feels right for me and is aligned with my values, beliefs and priorities, within 3 to 6 months of any redundancy.	Must ensure compatibility with beliefs and values; must have scope for making a real difference to people's lives, as well as aiding my professional progress
Medium-Term Goals	To engage in active networking, identifying key people who can help my job search	Evaluate after 3 months how many people I've identified and had direct communication with, through work contacts, courses or social events	Networking can be easily integrated into current job demands
	To embark on the next phase of my psychotherapy training, to add the next dimension to my skills and knowledge	Commence psychotherapy course at the beginning of autumn term	Some anxiety about accommodating course around new baby, but only 1 day per month, and easily accessible; comfortable about fitting private study around domestic demands
	To search through newspapers, websites and healthcare literature to develop a good understanding of the range of job options	Within 3 months to have compiled a list of organisations who could use my experience and skills, especially in quality and strategy management, and for whom I would feel happy working	Researching job options a natural consequence of current circumstances and career stage
Short-Term Goals	To update my CV	Update CV by the end of this month	No conflicts with CV – just need to identify appropriate references
	To write a business case proposing a new post with my current employer utilising and developing my current skills	To submit business proposal by the end of next month	Minimal dissonance with regard to business case – identifying new channels where my skills could be used to benefit the organisation

Figure 7.2   Goal setting process

The TGROW method

At this stage it might be useful to summarise the five stages that we have explored. They can be brought together under a specific model often used in coaching which forms the basis of an alternative, slightly more formalised method of self-coaching, or coaching of others, driven by this theme of goal setting. It is called the TGROW method. There are five steps to this process:

T – Theme (see the Wheel of Life Exercise in Chapter 4)

G – Goals (clear identification)

R – Reality (the ecology check as detailed earlier)

O – Options (checking out alternatives, making sure you have selected the best)

W – Will (evidence and actions in order to make a commitment)

The TGROW method can also be visualised as a learning model. This approach can be a great help during the process of goal setting, bringing together a number of coaching techniques in a condensed and easy to use mechanism.

This method can be used either alone or with others. In order for your time to be productive, it is suggested that you adhere to the specific process once you have identified which area or aspect of your life you wish to explore and change. Some examples might be your study habits, your domestic arrangements, or your career. The model is illustrated in Figure 7.3 below.

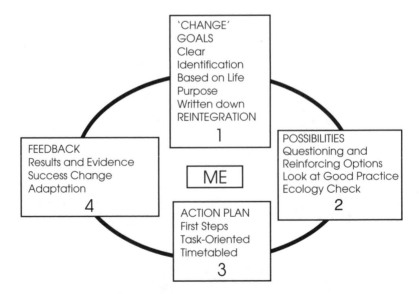

Figure 7.3 The TGROW model

We can amplify each of the headings in the illustration.

Goals

Goals affect all our performance, especially when they are based in our fundamental beliefs and values. This requires a clear analysis of any assumptions surrounding our goals in order that we select what we really want.

Possibilities

Begins with questioning and reflecting on identified goals and considering all options. Enabling strategies, such as the identification of good practice and role modelling, can support the realisation of goals and outcomes. This process also identifies the relevant resources that might be required. Finally, run an ecology check. Does it fit in with your wider life?

Action Plans

This involves identifying 'first steps' that are realistic and timetabled in order to deliver goals. Plans are supported by self-management techniques to bolster feedback and gear responses towards success and improvement.

Feedback

The feedback phase involves careful monitoring and response. It requires you to revisit original goals and reset new targets where relevant.

Exercise 7.4
A Self-Coaching Discussion Exercise

Ask a series of self-empowering questions

1.a **Where am I now in terms of my goals or outcomes?**
Offer factual statements – an overview.

1.b **What progress have I made to fulfil my goals?**
Specify content, responses, facts, figures, and any obstacles.

2.a **What do I intend to do to improve and move ahead?**
These plans should be realistic, within your control. What support or advice, if any, is needed?

2.b **What else is there in terms of the required resources?**
Have I got all the knowledge I require? Do I need to find any new skills, and if so how will I get them?

2.c Does the goal that I have identified suit my wider life?
Carry out an ecology check:
What will I get if I achieve it?
What will I not get if I achieve it?
What will I get if I do not achieve it?
What will I not get if I do not achieve it?

3.a What first steps will I take to begin the changes?
Devise a set of actions for each goal, starting with one clear step in
each case. Make sure the first step is clear and achievable.

3.b How will I know when I have achieved my goals?
What evidence and what criteria will I use to measure success?

3.c When will I carry out these actions?
Plan a clear timetable ahead of the next meeting.

4.a Measure success through feedback
Summarise my progress to date.

4.b Set new goals, or retain existing goals.

Identified Specific Goal	Options Meant for Reaching Goal	Action Plan Individual Targets Timetable	Recorded Evidence for Feedback	New Targets	New Action Plan

(A blank version of this table can be found on the website at www.wiley.com/go/
nlphealthcare)

Figure 7.4 Recording and monitoring progress

Summary – the enduring benefits of goal setting

To hit the bull's eye you need to aim slightly above it to allow for the weight of the arrow and the pull of gravity on its way to the target. Isn't that equally true in life? If we build in a plan for any setbacks and accept there will be obstacles and things which take us off our path, then we can achieve our goals. Set your sights high, you may be surprised at how easily you reach your target.

We have sought to define and describe the principle and practice involved in the discipline of goal setting. We have offered a set of tools to enable you to begin to utilise the skill that we all possess in this area to make the differences in our lives that we desire.

There is a criticism in some circles that the discipline of goal setting can become compulsive and an obsession. To counter this, there is a great deal of evidence to show that those people who are deemed as high achieving, in a wide variety of fields, set at the heart of their endeavours the desire to achieve specific goals, and possess the knowledge to do it effectively. Joe Simpson, in his book *Touching the Void*, describes how he managed to save his own life by setting hourly goals to ensure that he kept his mind focused when he was stranded on a mountain in hostile conditions. Miraculously, he was able to get himself down to safety, despite having broken a leg.

Whenever I am working with groups in healthcare settings, it is apparent that few people use the skill of goal setting in any meaningful and disciplined way. This could explain how ready and open they are to learning about it and trying to embrace it. Many people have described to me how dedicating themselves to a set of goals has transformed their lives both professionally and personally.

These same people who have successfully set goals often define their main obstacle as being the need to overcome the fear that, by committing themselves to goals, they are claiming to be 'something special', and somehow setting themselves up for failure or ridicule. Why become snared in the myth that undue self-effacement is somehow admirable? As Joseph O'Connor (2001, p. 11) observes, 'When you do not know what you want, there are many people who are only too delighted to set you to work getting *their* outcomes.' This is not simply some modern, one-eyed, 'go-getting' philosophy. As a character in Anthony Trollope's 1864 novel *The Small House at Allington* states, 'Never think that you're not good enough yourself. A man should never think that. My belief is that in life people will take you very much at your own reckoning.'

Most crucially, goal setting gives a structure to imagine and achieve the desired outcomes that we want to secure in our lives to make the difference. They are a way of plotting a route away from where we have become stuck towards where we ideally want to be. If they are linked to our wider vision, as described in this chapter, they can deliver us the results that fit in with our fundamental life values. Specifically, goals allow us to address the common issues that concern us: self-belief and confidence, our ability to be assertive and to get our needs met, to be effective at work and in our personal relations, and to manage our time and stress levels.

This might all be summarised within the debate about work/life balance. As the ecology checking principle demonstrates, there is little point in us rigidly pursuing our demanding careers being at work fourteen hours each day if it is going to negatively affect our family life. Goal setting enables us to ask some deeper questions of ourselves in order to remain balanced and yet stimulated by work, with the added guidance of a planned journey operated through clearly identified goals. Can you imagine achieving even more through the setting of meaningful goals? You will wonder how you managed without them, once they become part of your normal routine.

References

Andreas, S., Faulkener, C. (1994) *NLP: The new technology of achievement.* London, Nicholas Brealey.

Knight, S. (2002) *NLP at Work.* London, Nicholas Brealey Publishing.

Murphy, J. (1988) *The Power of Your Sub-Conscious Mind.* London, Simon and Schuster.

O'Connor J. (2001) *NLP Workbook.* London, Element.

Smart, J. www.Saladltd.co.uk

Simpson, J. (1998) *Touching the Void.* Colchester, Vintage.

Yeats, W.B. (1990) *Collected Poems of W.B. Yeats.* London, Picador Books.

Self-managing for results

8

Jim Lister

> Learning is sometimes like a light bulb going on; it has always been there but never lit up.

In the previous chapter we established how significant goals can be used in determining and achieving what it is we want to achieve in our lives. So how do we begin to turn these goals into concerted action that is based in what we believe will be secured success, at least as far as we can tell? This chapter will present the answers we require so that we can turn our goals into reality.

So far we have explored a number of different approaches to self-managing and coaching in order to foster self-belief, to encourage the independent management of our states, and to build self-confidence. These techniques will inevitably forge the changes you desire in yourself, in the direction that you intend to take your career, and in your working relationships. They will also support the way that you are managing any uncertainties and anxieties, and can help you to control the stress that can build inside when you are facing change or conflict, threatening to prevent you performing to your full potential. We now need to establish strategies for dealing with the fear element, or patterns of negative thinking which are perpetuated through limiting beliefs and damaging internal dialogue. All of these can have a huge effect when we deal with situations where we feel insecure, or where we are being asked to step outside of our comfort zones. Instead of escalating these negative states, can you imagine how much more powerful it would be to run a positive strategy where you knew you could succeed and achieve the outcome you desire?

So what specifically are these situations in which we can feel under unaccustomed or heightened stress or anxiety? In many ways, they are 'moments of truth' or defining incidents in our lives, when the real fibres of our character are tested, and we struggle to put our goals and ambitions into practice. To define these pivotal moments in such honest terms might seem to be simply exaggerating their potentially intimidating nature, but if we are to prepare for success in facing them, we need to be honest about their power and significance in shaping our lives and careers. And there is simply no need to be cowed and fearful when faced with these potentially defining moments in our lives. Armed with a new effective strategy for confronting them intelligently and courageously, we can actually use these events to employ the range of talents and resources at our disposal, demonstrating everything positive that we have to offer to ourselves, to our patients, colleagues, families and friends – and yes, even to our bosses!

Does it seem so unimaginable that the situations we would normally approach with dread ought in reality to be confronted with confident anticipation, even a sense of excited relish? If so, then think back to a time when you successfully faced a challenge, and achieved something that made you feel proud and fulfilled. Don't pretend you can't remember one, because we have all had them! It might have been an examination, an interview, a physical or sporting endeavour, or a social event. Can you recall the sense of assurance with which you went into the challenge, confident that all the necessary resources were in place for you? It might have just seemed that things happened to come together that day, for some inexplicable reason, but there was really a pattern behind your success, and that pattern can be captured so that you can use it again, whenever it would be beneficial to do so.

So think of this chapter as a sort of guide to brewing your own real ale, or creating a fine, delicious wine from home-grown grapes, only in this case you are fermenting self-confidence as a prelude to success. We will show you a way of distilling those essential ingredients so that you can negotiate every 'moment of truth' with the same formula for success that you have already used instinctively on many previous occasions. In short, this chapter will help you manage yourself to get the results you desire.

Moving towards our targets

So how do we get the results that we want, when faced by these challenges beyond our everyday tasks and responsibilities, in which we actually go about putting our goals and ambitions on the line? Some examples of these challenges might be:

- a job interview
- a personal, developmental review
- implementing a new technique

- a disciplinary meeting
- a restructure with new job responsibilities
- a feedback meeting with a manager or colleague
- delivering a difficult message to a colleague, face to face
- and, the most threatening of all for many people, public speaking

Customarily, when we are faced with these situations, we find ways of reinforcing the messages that we give ourselves internally that we will find the situation difficult, even impossible, that we are not good enough and that we will fail. Sure enough, during and afterwards, we have our doubts confirmed. This evidence then reinforces our negative opinion of ourselves for the next time, and we are caught in a cycle of low self-regard whenever it comes to dealing with these crucial moments in our professional and personal lives. We manage by getting through by the seat of our pants, or by dismissing failure as inevitable, and out of our control. We get what we ask for and we get what we focus on!

Would you like to start asking for something different? Can we consciously break these patterns? Or are they so deeply rooted that they cannot be challenged unless we rely on good fortune on the day of the interview or review? When we do succeed, must we assume that it was because the interviewers or reviewers seemed to be good people and things just clicked, or could we have planned it that way? Are we clear about why we succeed? Are you clear how you can ensure future success?

This chapter will outline a specific, conscious process which allows us to boost ourselves in these challenging situations, in order that we behave and respond in the way that we wish, to get the results that we want. It requires daily preparation leading up to the significant event, following a specific step-by-step process, and it takes practice in order to make it work for you. We've called it the '4 Step Self-Manager Formula', and it pulls together a number of the techniques explored elsewhere in this book, applies them in a new way and also introduces some new concepts which can be effectively used alongside them, for a complete package which will allow you to ensure excellent, positive results.

The '4 Step Self-Manager Formula' for your future success

The four steps are as follows:

1. Set your goal, what it is you want to achieve in that situation, on that day, in that specific event, such as a meeting or interview or presentation, or even

just on one particularly demanding day of work. Be absolutely clear of the outcome you want to achieve, and focus on it.

2. Identify all the inner resources that you will need to reach your goal or target.

3. Think back to when you have achieved similar goals before in your life, and anchor these moments in your mental preparation.

4. Mentally rehearse, through future pacing, the event or challenge that you are about to encounter.

We will now look in detail at how to undertake each separate step, and then we will bring all of the steps together in a case study that applies the whole formula.

Step 1. Identify your goal or target

As Chapter 7 explores in depth, a clear identification and statement of our primary goal or target is the essential starting point. Stated as a positive outcome, that is what you want to achieve, not what you do not want to achieve, identified as achievable and realistic, within our control, and in line with our core values and beliefs, the goal will begin to drive all our actions and behaviours so that we achieve what it is we want.

Everything that you require in order to set about constructively setting your goals is outlined in Chapter 7, and it is important that you thoroughly recall and digest these approaches before going on any further into this 4 Step Self-Manager Formula.

The types of goal setting statement that you might establish are:

- It is March 2008 and I have contributed positively by expressing my opinion in four consecutive team meetings.

- It is December 2009 and I have communicated to my manager what I believe is the best way forwards for the organisation and especially for our department.

- It is April 2008 and I have given a clear direction to Anna, a member of my staff, in order that she will feel newly motivated to enable her to look at ways to improve her performance within the next three months.

This clarity of thinking, by considering and then stating exactly what we want and by when, is a critical starting point. In the experience of many people teaching the use of NLP, it is often underestimated and given too little thought. We encourage you to follow the goal setting processes outlined earlier in this book, and be rigorous in deciding what it is you want, guided by the golden rules of goal setting (Chapter 7).

Step 2. Identify the resources you need to reach your goal

Having identified both the direction you want to go in and your eventual destination, what exactly will you need to get you there and to maintain that direction despite the various setbacks, difficulties and unknowns that will inevitably occur en route to your success? The tools for the job can be defined as your resources, and we'd like to take you through a specific format in order for you to identify the critical resources required. You might also like to look at Chapter 9, which explores what energises you, as you may be able to utilise this to further enhance your resources.

Our resources

The resources that we will discuss in this context can be divided into three categories:

1. Beliefs
2. Behaviours
3. Actions

These three areas are inter-dependent, enhancing each other for maximum effectiveness. Let us start with the deeper level of beliefs.

1. Beliefs

Again, you might like to refer back to Chapter 5 on values and beliefs to remind yourself of your own values and beliefs in a work context. Start to ask yourself again here, what beliefs do I need to have, crucially and as a first priority, in order to achieve my goal? They might be to do with yourself, your inner self-belief, or faith in your technical ability to carry out the task in hand. It might be belief in your abilities as a learner, a manager, a supportive colleague, or a friend. In order to answer this question you might also find it helpful to ask another question: in which role or roles will I be required to operate in order to achieve my goal?

The more specific you can be in identifying your beliefs, the more you will be able to pinpoint where you have used or exhibited these qualities previously. This is a vital part of the next phase of the 4 Step Self-Manager Formula. It is not always easy to identify belief resources, as they are hidden from other people (we rarely talk about them) as well as from our own awareness (we rarely consider them). So a starting point is to consider the role you will be in, mentor, adviser, manager, disciplinarian, confidant, friend, and connect the empowering beliefs to that primary role. What is true about you in that role or more specifically, what has to be true about you in that role to do a fantastic job?

Here is a specific example of this within a role you might need to adopt. Imagine that you are about to present a report to a team of managers. Your primary role is as a presenter, but you might also be required to act as a negotiator and listener. The core beliefs you might therefore identify are:

> To believe in my own abilities to speak clearly and succinctly
>
> To believe I have sufficient knowledge to answer questions on the report
>
> To believe in my ability to receive feedback and respond to it positively
>
> To believe in my inner strength to stand in front of people and appear confident
>
> To believe in my ideas and in the practical suggestions that I am about to present
>
> To believe in the process that I am about to undertake in order to present my case.

2. Behaviours

Having identified the primary beliefs that we require in order to achieve the goal we have set ourselves, we can now turn to the next level of behaviours. Ask yourself the following question, 'How do I wish to behave during the pursuit of my goal?'

Do not be afraid to state the obvious. If we use the example above, my behaviours might be stated as:

- To conduct myself throughout the presentation calmly and with dignity
- To be open and accepting to feedback no matter what is offered
- To enjoy the presentation and introduce humour where appropriate
- To demonstrate that I have prepared thoroughly for the presentation
- To be passionate about what it is I am saying and to show that I believe in the ideas and in the benefits of what I am suggesting
- To be spontaneous

3. Actions

Having answered how I intend to be, I now need to look at what I intend to do, in order to achieve my goal. Using the same example once again, my actions can be listed as follows:

- To have cleaned my shoes and have a handkerchief or tissue
- To arrive on time, or slightly early to put things in place
- To drink water throughout
- To have turned off my mobile phone
- To stand as still as possible
- To have a deliberate slow, calm delivery in my voice as I speak
- To tell at least two jokes at the appropriate moment
- To give eye contact to everyone in the room wherever possible
- To ask questions rather than simply give answers

Once you have begun to list the actions you require, then the more detailed they tend to become. The possibilities are endless and you will find that your action list starts to become very long. Take your time and enjoy exploring the detail with a thoroughness you might never have thought possible regarding one single event. Be surprised at how many of them seem very 'doable' to you, acknowledging how far you have already come to reaching your goals.

A process for identifying vital resources

In this Self-Manager Formula the identification of our key resources is vital. It is an area that we often fail to consider or spend time preparing for. We leave it to our subconscious to present what we need on the day and in the very moment of the event. However, as we have seen, our subconscious needs guidance and a direct message or command in order for it to be focused and responsive to the specific nature of a potentially stressful or challenging situation.

The resources that we possess are unlimited, once we start to really understand ourselves. Think of any situation that you might find potentially difficult, and it will soon become clear how you wish to go about dealing with this, what you have to do in practice, and in which areas you need to believe. These insights working together offer us greater reassurance that we can go about achieving our goal, easily and effectively and they give both a conscious and subconscious set of messages that guide us as we set about the task.

Before moving on to the next step, it is worth spending a little more time looking at how we can identify and discover our resources and pinpoint the most significant ones we require.

It is necessary to consult your subconscious, and to do this it is essential to commit yourself to a deeper level of thinking rather than approaching this task as a conscious, logical or intellectual process. Therefore, you will need to sit in a quiet place where you are able to concentrate without disturbance. Sit in a restful position with your hands in your lap, and with your eyes closed.

Exercise 8.1
Making Your Goals a Reality

First of all, listen to your own breathing, and become focused on hearing your own breath as it goes in and out. Gradually begin to exclude any other thoughts, breathe out any negative emotion or tension with each breath and breathe in a feeling of strength and confidence. After a short while, consider your clearly stated goal. Ask yourself, 'What resources will I need in order to achieve this goal?'

Then ask yourself what practical actions you will need to take. Allow your subconscious to present all the answers it can. Don't question or block whatever enters your mind. You are conducting a subconscious search so allow the process to unfold, and be surprised at how much you uncover.

Secondly, carry out the same process with regard to your behaviours by asking how you will need to behave. And allow yourself to be surprised at what emerges.

Finally, ask yourself what beliefs you need in order to carry out and achieve your goal. What beliefs will empower you? Which ones are essential and go to the heart of the matter that you are dealing with?

Having spent between 10 and 15 minutes on this process, allow yourself to re-emerge into your fully conscious state, become aware of your surroundings and slowly pick up your pen again and get ready to write. Go about writing down the key actions, behaviours and beliefs that have emerged so far. You will now have a clear set of resources that you know will be required to achieve your goal. The next step simply asks you to identify where and when you have used the same kinds of resources before in your life, in order to prove that, if you have done similar things before, you can certainly do them again even more effectively, each time you use these resources you will find that you can access them more quickly and use them more powerfully to get the results you want.

The importance of identifying and preparing our resources

Before we move on to the next step, called anchoring, it is worth reaffirming why it is so essential that we prepare our resources in this way.

All of our actions, behaviours and beliefs are learned through our life's experiences. The more we are exposed to those situations in which we feel uneasy, the more we are likely to trigger the usual, expected responses within ourselves. We almost encourage ourselves to struggle with the challenges of the situation, and the evidence just keeps mounting to prove that this is how it is and always will be! It is rather like pressing a button in our mind to run the old familiar programme, which we may not like, but which we at least understand and own.

In this section of the book, we are presenting a tool that will help you break the chain, and allow yourself to take possession of what you want. However, it means learning some new ways, and unlearning the old, more established routines, which can be deeply rooted and hard to throw off without knowing the right tools to use. In order to do this you will need discipline and determination, and some of your most precious resource: quality time. In the end, it will be up to you, aided by the kind of framework that is offered in this chapter. How much do you really want to make the change?

Step 3. Anchors

Anchoring is the technique of recalling a positive 'state' through a memory of an experience and replaying it in the mind. An anchor acts as a trigger to becoming more resourceful when we replay this state and use it whenever we choose. It allows you to create in yourself any chosen 'state' at will. It is particularly useful when we want to be more in control in a difficult situation.

The anchors that exist within us all are many and varied, and they each have a specific trigger that fires the anchor inside us to come alive. Think of the word holiday, and you will probably start to fill up with a warm feeling of well-being! The trigger is the actual word holiday, and the specific anchor could be any holiday you have experienced which has brought you pleasure and enjoyment. It would seem sensible to choose the one that you enjoyed most! Equally, listen to your favourite piece of music, and similar feelings will emerge. The notes of the music will provide the first trigger, and the anchor is probably a mixture of the sheer beauty of the music and the associated memories and feelings that you attach to it, where you were when you first heard it, who you were with, what you were doing, etc.

Bear in mind that we have both positive and negative anchors. A certain piece of music might bring up negative connotations and memories. Our feelings here could be melancholic. Equally, if someone asks you to wash the dishes, these words probably trigger negative anchors, which encourage you to move away from doing the task, rather than lovingly embracing it. It is possible that when you think of doing a certain task, or you recall a certain person, you can trigger negative feelings inside you, but don't dwell on them, think again of a positive anchor, one which uplifts you and makes you feel good about yourself.

It is worth just considering some of the anchors your patients may have associated with the hospital. For example if a patient is receiving ongoing treatment, a door to a department, or a particular smell, or a uniform may trigger a negative state in them, without them even being aware of the internal processes which are occurring. How empowering would it be for them, to help them generate positive anchors to help them to create a positive state while in your care? While we are exploring the use of anchoring here within self-management, it is worth thinking through other applications for you and your patients, colleagues and friends. Just take a few moments and write down other potential uses of anchoring in your own practice and life.

So, in the context of self-management, how do we use this day-to-day technique of anchoring that already exists everywhere in our lives, to bolster our ability to achieve the work-related goal we have set ourselves? Clearly, we want to activate positive anchors rather than negative ones.

Start by running through your mind the key resources that you have already identified during Step 2. Choose by prioritising no more than four or five of them. Once you have done this, think back to a time when you have used each of these resources successfully, perhaps without realising it at the time. Preferably it will be in a similar situation and in the pursuit of a similar goal. However, if you cannot locate a direct comparison, it is still very useful to identify a particular situation in which you have used these resources in the past, or even to imagine what it would be like if you had used them effectively, as your unconscious mind does not distinguish between real and imagined feelings. By doing this you are beginning to locate your anchor. Once you have located your anchor, work through Exercise 8.2 below to build that anchor into a positive resource you can use whenever you need it.

How to build an anchor

Before you work through Exercise 8.2, we suggest that you read through the whole section. Become familiar with it, and then read it again and begin to apply it to build your own anchor.

Exercise 8.2
Anchoring

Sit in a quiet space in which you can concentrate in a similar way to what you did in the earlier 'resource identification' exercise. Start to search for that positive memory, when you can recall using these key resources. It might be from an event that happened the other week, it might be from a year ago, or it might be from 5, 10, or 35 years ago! The important thing is that it fits the following essential criteria:

- It has to bring out wholly positive associations within you rather than negative emotions such as sadness or regret
- It has to be something you want to recall
- It has to feature you as a central character
- It has to have a clear location that can be seen in your mind's eye
- It has to bring back strong, positive feelings when you recall it

Once you have conducted the search of your subconscious memory bank, and are confident and happy that you have located that key moment or recollection, simply enjoy reliving it, in as much detail as you possibly can. As you rerun this film from your past, deepen your emotional engagement with your memory by contemplating these three questions:

- Firstly, 'What can I see in this film? What are the colours, movements, textures, locations, people?' Fill in as much detail as possible. Recall the perspective and the depth, the focus, the brightness of the colours, the shapes. It is rather like scanning a picture that you have chosen to look at, which gives great pleasure. You are seeking to take in as much detail as possible into the mind's eye, even more detail than you were aware you had initially recorded.
- Secondly, 'What sounds can I detect within the film? Are there environmental sounds, voices, or just unidentified, random noises?' Ask yourself what you can hear, what is the quality of the sound like, what variety, what volume? Where is the sound located, is it continuous or broken, near or far, clear or muffled? Again you are seeking as much detail as possible in your mind's ear.
- Thirdly, 'What qualities of feelings are associated with this film? Does the recollection make me feel happy, content, warm, smooth or sharp? And where are these feelings located in my body? Do those feelings have a colour or a shape? Are they moving or still?' Fill in as much detail as you possibly can by exploring how the film subtly affects your emotions.

These three primary, sensory responses, what we see (visual), what we hear (auditory) and what we feel (kinaesthetic), make up our experience of any event. The more we can rediscover these sensory responses, the more we can relocate the experience and reconnect with the resources that we used, in our 'successful' memory.

Triggering or firing our anchors

Once you have recollected the three sensory experiences, bring them all together and as powerfully as you can, associate into the past experience as if you are reliving it. Take your time and enjoy it. Intensify all the details so that the images and sounds are as compelling as possible. When you get to a point where you feel that you are fully associated, as if it is actually happening now, where you are experiencing it afresh, then either think of a word or a sound, or see a moment or object in your mind, or touch a particular point on yourself, for example touch your thumb and middle finger together on one hand quite firmly, and use this movement as your trigger. Hold it to a count of five, when the intensity of the feeling will begin to dissipate and then begin to relax and let go of your anchor.

The anchor is the positive state which you are capturing and the trigger is how you will access, or fire, that anchor in the future.

Testing your anchor

Let go completely of the past memory which you have been re-living and 'break your state'. Look at something in your room completely unrelated to the experience and stare at it for ten seconds. Stand up and turn around: do a 360 degree turn. Sit down, close your eyes and re-fire your anchor by triggering the thought, word, image or feeling/touch. Can you retrieve the association into that memory as powerfully as you did before? Do you notice how you just experience again that state easily and effortlessly?

Keep repeating this process as often as you can; if you have other memories which use similar feelings, then use those too, use memories which cover all the resources you identified as required. The more that you re-fire (or stack) and trigger the anchor and associate into it, the more you will build it into your automatic recall system, and the easier it will be to recall it as and when you need it. It will start to serve you as a clear reminder that you are capable of achieving your goal, and it will replace the doubts and the negative anchors that have historically blocked your progress.

Each time you believe or sense that you are fully in the moment of your anchor, at the peak, then apply a word or phrase, or a specific touch to reinforce your association. When you re-fire your anchor, repeat the word phrase or touch to help your recall.

You can continue to stack your anchor in the days and months ahead. Whenever you use the required resources and feel really good about how you have used them, fire your anchor again to build an even greater response tool for when you need it.

When you have mastered the technique consider building other anchors, for example one for calm and relaxed, one for happy and content. You might like to create one for confident, fluent and respected to use during presentations. Make sure each anchor has a unique and specific trigger. A good tip is to use a trigger which is not likely to be set off unintentionally. Also consider how practical the trigger is, for example, holding your left toe is not appropriate as a trigger for an anchor for presenting. Remember your specific anchors for each state and use them to achieve your desired state whenever you want to feel a certain way. Use your anchors to help you to achieve your desired results.

The benefits of anchoring

I invariably cover this skill of anchoring whenever I am working with people in healthcare settings. Groups usually grasp the principle quickly, and after we have run at least two new anchors and taken the group through the complete sequence described earlier, participants find that they have been helped into a significant state change. In the longer term, this technique offers people greater confidence, a calm realisation that they can indeed succeed in a challenge. They realise that, after all, they have done it or something like it before. Nearly everyone I work with says how pleasing it is to rediscover an episode from their lives that they'd forgotten. It produces evidence that our subconscious can give us all that we need providing it is guided, and the key resources are asked for.

Most importantly, the vital skill of anchoring proves to us that we are capable and accomplished, and that we are justified in being self-confident. This in turn produces a deeper self-belief to get us through the journey to achieving our goals. As one workshop participant who attended a training day held by the College of Radiographers in London memorably stated on the feedback sheet: 'On the anchoring technique – I've never thought of doing that – and wow!'

It might help to guide you in this process to pause for a moment and consider how a fellow healthcare professional aided her effectiveness at work, and indeed significantly boosted her career, firstly by defining key resources she would need to face a demanding situation, and then using these resources to build an anchor.

Diana's Story

A colleague was hampering my ability to do my job by her aggressive and intimidating behaviour in strategy meetings and working groups. She appeared to take pleasure in provoking disagreement, and didn't seem happy unless she was in the thick of an argument. I started experiencing strong feelings of anxiety, and a sick feeling in the pit of my stomach, whenever a conflict was about to erupt. I used to cave in to her straight away, without expressing my point of view, just to avoid disputes and bad feeling.

I used this experience when we were covering the technique of anchoring on an NLP course. I discovered that the resources I needed to become more effective during these moments of confrontation were confidence and self-belief. I recalled an incident two years previously when I had displayed these qualities, and I 'transported' myself back there to relive as vividly as possible what it was like, where I was, what I could see, smell and hear, what it actually felt like to experience and show these resources. I developed a small tactile gesture to summon up those resources again when I needed them.

The very act of reminding myself that I possessed these reserves of character helped no end. During the next working group, when my colleague began provoking an argument, I calmed myself by breathing deeply, checked my posture, faced her square on, and fired my self-belief anchor. Having re-ignited what it was like to display those qualities, I felt composed and under control, and I argued my case clearly and persuasively.

I combined this use of anchoring with some perceptual positioning work (Chapter 6), and began to realise that, as my colleague came from an academic background, vigorous debate was simply her way of establishing the best course of action. What I had seen as conflict and bad feeling was to her healthy debate, and I began to appreciate that the working group was all the more dynamic and effective as a result of that.

We had never actually been on bad terms, and we are now close friends. One of my goals at the time had been to become more assertive during group strategy meetings, and to express my views more persuasively. I feel that the first time I stood up effectively to my forthright colleague was a key moment in my career, and I know that I can reinstate and rely on those resources of self-belief and confidence in any similar situation from now on.

Step 4. Mental rehearsal

The only way to ensure you get the future you want is to create it now. In following the three steps detailed so far, goal setting, identifying resources, and establishing positive anchors, we have allowed ourselves to enjoy quality time in our preparation and to take positive thoughts into our journey. Hopefully, we have successfully reached the destination of achieving our goal. One final preparation exercise will help reinforce the advantage that we have created for ourselves so far. It is often referred to as 'visualisation' and we'd like you to explore an extended version so that you can plot or pace your future by running a thorough mental rehearsal of what you intend to do.

How to mentally rehearse

Again, a prerequisite to achieving the most substantial benefits from this technique is a quiet undisturbed space where you can concentrate for between 10 and 20 minutes.

Exercise 8.3
Mental Rehearsal (1)
(There is a second mental rehearsal exercise in Chapter 9)

The starting point is to create images in your mind's eye, envisioning the things that you wish to achieve in this 'pivotal' or significant encounter, from start to finish. Begin with the start of your journey in as much detail as possible. Where will you begin? Who else is involved? What do you intend to do, and how will you do it through the behaviours identified in Step 2?

You are seeking to build a logical programme, episode by episode, from the start of your journey through until your final destination and the achievement of your goal. See yourself starting from the place where you begin and create the movie in your mind. As you move through the episodes, focus on key moments, the ones that are more likely to be problematic or difficult. See, hear and feel yourself managing to overcome any of the hurdles which might present themselves, by taking the action you intend, in the way that you intend, using all the resources now available to yourself. Lastly, see, hear and feel the final point of achievement, where you get exactly the result you want, in the way you want it. Be clear about how you will know your goal has been met, know what you will see, hear or feel, and focus on that desired outcome.

Mental rehearsal should follow a 'time line' from the present into the future (see p. 168). Go along this time line at whatever pace you desire, or at a pace that suits the process. Fill in as much detail as you can – where, when, who and how – and see, hear and feel as much as possible. I have known people spend over an hour preparing in this way for a simple meeting. It is crucial that you envisage as many options, possibilities and outcomes as you can at any point on the time line. It is also worth including how you will cope with any deviations from the plan, so that if the rehearsal does not directly mirror the actual experience, you are not put off by any changes.

While you may not be able to envisage each specific potential deviation or obstacle, you can rehearse how you will deal with unexpected incidents, so that you have effectively covered all eventualities (see p. 165 for notes on putting a recovery strategy in place).

Here is how Susan used this technique to prepare for an important interview.

Susan's Story

Since leaving school, I had worked in a series of fairly low-key jobs. My levels of confidence were lower than they had ever been, and I had got into a rut of feeling as though I wasn't any good at anything. I got an interview for a demanding job that I really wanted. I knew I had the ability to do this job well, and it would have been a real turning point for me if I'd got it. But I was dreading the interview. I couldn't help telling myself, 'You can't do interviews, you're rubbish at this.' The thought of facing the interview was making me feel really low.

I decided to go to a coach to give me some tips on how to cope with the interview. I didn't have any great hopes for this, and I saw it as a bit of a last resort really. But the first thing we did made me feel better straight away. The coach asked me to say where I felt the anxiety about the interview, and I said in my stomach, so she asked me to say what colour it was, and to think of it as a ball of wool. Then she suggested I change its colour, and spin it away from my stomach, then roll it back in. It turned from an orange ball of anxiety into a blue one, and when I rolled the ball back in again, the anxiety had eased off!

The coach then asked me what had happened to give me these negative beliefs about myself. I couldn't help getting tearful, and I said I just got overcome with nerves when I was under pressure. I said how I felt I'd wasted my schooling, and had let my parents down in everything I'd tried to do. Though I was only in my early twenties, I felt I had been capable of much more, and had already thrown away all the chances I would have.

The coach listened, and then began to explain about the importance of giving myself positive messages. She described the effect my beliefs were having on my behaviour, and explained how my inner dialogue was setting me up to fail. She helped me to realise that I had a choice, to carry on giving in to the things causing this unhelpful behaviour, or to help myself into a more preferable state.

She then introduced me to an anchoring exercise, and I remembered back to a time a short while earlier just on a night out, nothing special, when I had felt great, and had not been worried or anxious about anything. I felt again what it was like to feel that good, and the coach explained how I could summon up that feeling again any time I wanted. She then took me on what she called a time line into the future. I had to imagine my interview was taking place, but I was hovering above it, watching myself performing confidently and success-fully. I then had to go down into the interview, being myself, imagining every detail of what it was like to be feeling happy and in control, to see exactly what it felt like. I ran through the stages of the interview, and rehearsed and practised what I would say, and how I would feel.

The coaching had a remarkable effect. On the day of the interview, I was able to use the techniques to control my nerves, and I felt at ease, and totally assured during the questioning. I just felt that I was the right person for the job, and the interviewers must have agreed, as they appointed me to the post!

A recovery strategy

I am often asked what happens to us when reality doesn't turn out quite as we had imagined it might during our mental rehearsal. How do we prepare for the unknown, which will almost inevitably occur, something that we had failed to consider in our mental preparation? My answer is to prepare for this by mentally rehearsing your recovery from anything that might throw you off course.

For example, if I am presenting an idea to a team of people, I can mentally rehearse the presentation by picturing the room, the people in it, what I am going to say, and how I want to say it. I can rehearse my state, and I can hear the tone of my voice. But I cannot imagine all of the responses to my presentation. I can imagine some of them, those who enthuse, those who doubt, but what if someone laughs in an unexpected place? What if the fire alarm goes off half-way through the session and we all end up standing in the rain for half an hour before coming back to finish off? The possibilities are endless and unknown. However, I can prepare myself by mentally rehearsing my recovery and response to the unknown. I can anticipate the way I wish to feel, and I can imagine the internal dialogue I might use in order to reassure myself and establish a mood of calmness in me and hopefully everyone else in the room.

Mental rehearsal is therefore a projection into the future of how we would like things to be. It would be great if this then automatically delivered the results we might want, without problems, consistently every time. Life is of course not like this. We know it will present the unknown. So we can prepare for that, and enact a strategy that allows us to take the fear out of the journey we are undertaking. The more that we can see, hear and feel success in our mental preparation, the more it is likely to happen. The only thing to lose is a small amount of time and the potential benefits are enormous.

The formula in action

The 4 Step Self-Manager Formula can now be pieced together. Although each stage is self-standing and will deliver benefits if used on its own, the combination of the steps acts in a 'super-additive' way, so that the total effect is greater than the sum of the individual parts. Below we present Marianne's story which illustrates how the formula was used in its entirety to deliver her goal. She took control of a very difficult situation for herself. She admitted that she had thought that it would have been easier to ignore it or to leave the job.

Marianne's Story

Marianne managed a palliative care team of 22 people across three districts. The team rarely had the chance to meet as one unit, and whenever they did manage to meet up the members stated how useful it was. Unfortunately, it became apparent that sessions were starting to be dominated by two powerful members, who were known to each other and were highly competitive. They played out their power struggle in front of the rest of the team, and despite a variety of attempts to steer matters in another direction, things always ended up the same, with two senior people in disagreement, using the team meeting to try and settle their own personal scores. This inevitably damaged the morale of the other team members.

Marianne knew that she had to take action. She was relatively new in post. She had been an internal appointment, and had worked under both of the individuals in her earlier career. She knew them both well, and they knew her. Up to now, neither had been particularly responsive to her management style, and Marianne felt her confidence was being undermined, and her enthusiasm started ebbing away. However, she knew that if she could address the two people directly, then she would begin to re-establish herself and assert her credibility as a new manger, in everyone's eyes. Marianne knew she had to show real leadership otherwise she might never regain her authority or the confidence of her team members.

The rest of the story is in Marianne's words.

I felt genuinely afraid of taking on this situation and managing it. I thought they'd just ignore me and treat me like a junior, just like they did when I worked for them. Every time I thought about it I just froze, just didn't want the task. It made me lose sleep and start to wish I hadn't taken the job. I started to wake up feeling sick in the morning, dreading going into work.

I attended one of your workshops organised through my employer, and thought I'd try and put your ideas into practice, step by step.

First of all, I set out my goal. The irony was that I was very clear about what it was I wanted to achieve. I wanted to set up individual meetings with each person, and then bring both of them together to clear the air, let each other hear one another's problems, and then establish a new way forward, with me as their manager, one which they would both sign up to. It sounded so easy, but I just didn't feel that I had the confidence to do it.

I sat down and started to identify the resources that I would need. I kept coming up with courage, clear thinking, authority and a clear plan. All sorts of other resources would flash through my mind, but it was these qualities that seemed essential. I probably thought about it four or five times over a few days.

I decided to try and anchor these qualities, especially courage. Whilst I relaxed and thought, I found that I'd done many things in my life, especially when I was travelling, which had involved me being very strong and coura-geous. Maybe those occasions involved different circumstances, but they still made me reveal the qualities I now wanted to show in dealing with my two col-leagues. I suppose I set up at least three anchors. One especially strong anchor was triggered by the phrase 'I can do this, anytime any place!'

I called them to meetings the following week, and mentally rehearsed for each one. They went like a dream for me, and we got to where I hoped we would. I think they were surprised how strong I seemed, and how clear I was about what was wanted. I made sure they each had plenty of time to speak, and then to listen to me.

After that, I kept up my approaches with them. I think they know where they stand with me now, and I've got them to address the real problems that had never properly been spoken about. I was and still am amazed at how I handled it and the results I got, for all three of us and for the wider team, which has greatly improved. It has really boosted my confidence in my ability to manage difficult situations that crop up between people.

The four stages shown in the formula allowed me to have a structure for my preparation. I'd never really thought about it before. I'd just been turning up to work, and ended up dealing with situations, like a fire fighter, reacting whenever a problem came up. I'm now much more able to plan, prepare and feel confident I'll sort things out whenever they occur. It has been a bit of a revelation for me. I know I can manage people now. I spend some time every week sticking with the ideas and practising the techniques so that I'm achieving what I want.

Using time lines

We mentioned the use of time lines as part of your mental rehearsal. Using time lines is an incredibly useful way of both revisiting things from the past and also looking at how things will be in the future. All our memories are stored, albeit unconsciously, in an orderly fashion so that they can be retrieved. For example you can tell the difference easily between a journey you did yesterday and one you did last year. One way of storing memories is in time sequence.

Just take a moment and think about something you did last week. Where in relation to you is that experience? Is it to your left or is it behind you? Now think of something that you know will happen in the future, a holiday you have planned, or an event you are looking forward to. Where is that in relation to where you are? Is it to your right or in front of you? People tend to have one of two patterns in respect of time lines: in time and through time (Figure 8.1).

It is useful to know where your time line is for a number of reasons. Time Line Therapy™ (developed by Tad James) is a powerful therapy for eliminating negative emotions such as anger, sadness, fear and guilt and can also be used to remove limiting beliefs, such as 'I am not good enough', 'I am hopeless', which if left untreated will impact hugely on your ability to achieve your full potential as

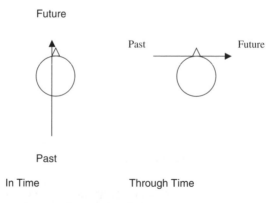

Figure 8.1 Where the experience is in relation to you

it is your beliefs that determine your behaviour. If this is something that interests you find yourself a qualified Time Line Therapy coach to work through those issues with you. Time Line Therapy is a dissociated, safe technique which quickly removes obstacles which have inhibited you for many years, possibly without you even realising the negative effect they were having. While we cannot go into the potential change interventions here, as you require qualified support to undertake that work, we can share with you the use of a basic time line which can be of enormous benefit when setting goals.

Exercise 8.4
Using Your Time Line

In the context of mental rehearsal if you take a few moments to float up above your time line, just close your eyes and relax and see yourself below on your time line, see your past stretching behind (or to the left of) you and your future stretching out in front (or to your right). You will find that this is a very calm and safe place to be and you might find this is a useful relaxation method for you which you can use in its own right. For this exercise, just take a few moments to drift back above your past, see some of the great times you have had, stay well up above your time line over any unhappy times to avoid getting re-associated with any negative feelings and drop into any great times to re-experience your positive emotions. Turn around and drift forward, moving again over the present time. Keep moving forward and now drift out into your future. Drift forward to a time when you will use your mental rehearsal, a specific time, and take a compelling picture of how you want that event to be and drop it very deliberately at the right point in your future time line. Make the picture big and bright and lock it into position so it will be there when you need it. You can even go beyond that time and feel how good things are, with that picture in place when your goal has been met and you successfully used those resources, before floating pack to the present time and coming back down into the here and now.

As we said before, this technique is also useful for putting goals into your time line, giving extra compulsion to any time-setting component of the goals you set in Chapter 7. Take some time now to put your goals in your future time line using this technique, they will act as a magnet drawing you towards them. Make the pictures of each goal really compelling, imagine yourself having achieved that goal. What will you see, what will you hear and what will you feel? Imagine you have already attained that goal and feel the emotion attached to achieving it. Then take that picture to the appropriate point in the future and lock it into your time line, so your subconscious has a clear message about when to achieve the goal by.

Summary

This chapter has brought together four individual techniques and unified them as one process, designed to help us exploit the skills and talents we already possess to prepare for the kinds of challenging situations that we all must inevitably encounter at key points in our lives. These techniques have been placed in an order that progresses naturally from one to the other, so that you may get the result you desire:

Goal setting, resource identification, anchoring, mental rehearsal.

The strategies require mental preparation and time. However, this investment of time and effort, often carried out the day before, or as in Marianne's case, the week before, can give great returns, especially in our self-belief. What might have seemed difficult, impossible, threatening or frightening now seems surprisingly manageable and deliverable because we have chosen to take responsibility for ourselves, using the tools that will enable us to self-manage through the clear, tangible framework offered by this simple formula. And the main resource we need is actually in plentiful supply, the wisdom we have already accumulated from our past experiences.

How good is it to know that we already have everything we need within ourselves and this formula will help us to identify and access those resources. Can you imagine being able to access those resources whenever they are required? With practice you will be surprised just how easy this is to achieve.

A final metaphor might help to reinforce the value of integrating the techniques in this toolkit regularly and consistently into your working practices and daily routines. As stated in the introduction to the chapter, the tools will prove especially useful for overcoming those 'pivotal' challenges that we all have to face at times, when our lives reach a crucial intersection or crossroads. Negotiating a complicated road junction we have never encountered before can lead to unbridled confusion and panic, all kinds of hand flapping and neck twisting, wild-eyed staring at the bewildering array of signs and arrows, random, last-minute tugs at the steering wheel, wrong turnings, close scrapes, acrimony and recrimination, often culminating in torrid outbursts of profane language. Sounds familiar?

But have you noticed how these potential 'Spaghetti Junctions' pass by, provoking nothing more than a glow of satisfied achievement, when we have anticipated their approach, prepared for them in advance, familiarised ourselves with the road map, and recalled how we have in fact successfully negotiated them before? Don't the crucial intersections in our lives deserve to be met with the same level of care and foresight? Carry your NLP toolkit around with you, and we feel sure that you will notice a marked improvement in your driving wherever you are heading, and you can start to really enjoy the ride!

Overcoming hurdles and maintaining momentum

9

Liz Holland

> You can choose to accept things as they are and continue to get the results you are currently getting, or you can make a decision to change and not be held back by obstacles you encounter.

By now you will have done all the exercises and developed your goals. Now you are ready to go out and make your dreams a reality. Have you been in this position before? Have you in the past set goals which you have not kept? This chapter will give you all that you require to ensure that you invest time and energy into yourself, to care for yourself and to achieve all that you have set out to achieve.

One of the challenges for healthcare professionals is that our work can overtake our lives (see Chapter 4). For those employed in services that are provided 24 hours a day, 7 days a week, regular routines may be difficult to establish with changing rosters or being 'on call' and being required to be available at short notice. Healthcare professionals are frequently passionate about their work, and accept that being available to care for their patients is one of the major components of their work. Some may put their patients' needs above their own at times, yet unless we care for ourselves we will not be able to continue to care for others.

So what are some of the potential hurdles facing healthcare professionals today? Common themes identified include:

financial constraints

compliance with controls introduced by Government/registering bodies

high expectations of healthcare professionals from patients

fear of making mistakes

fear of litigation

lack of sleep for staff covering 24-hour rosters, despite employment laws that
may limit working hours

staff shortages

conflict between demands of career and personal life

increased paperwork and targets to meet

This chapter provides you with some practical ideas to assist you in overcoming
hurdles that you may encounter. The tools presented will assist you in:

1. managing your energy levels
2. identifying problems and what is causing them
3. managing stressful situations

As you read the activities and client stories think how you could apply the concepts to improve the quality of your own life and work.

1. Managing your energy levels

Time and energy can be resources that are in short supply for healthcare professionals. The demands of work, complicated and constantly changing organisations, running a business, working with people who are unwell and increasing
paperwork can all sap energy, leaving less for the professional and personal goals
that you have set for yourself.

To assist in overcoming time and energy-draining obstacles, it is important
to know what activities energise and revitalise you, and what activities sap you
of energy. Fortunately, we are all different, so what one person may find tedious
and energy-sapping another may find satisfying. By knowing ourselves, we can
maintain our energy by either deleting draining activities or by delegating them
to others who find them energising.

Coach U, a virtual university (see note, p. 198), has a Personal Foundation
Programme that includes very practical exercises. 'Zap the Tolerations' identifies
things that we put up with in life that distract us or sap our energy. By identifying
and acknowledging these tolerations you can stop trying to manage situations
that drain your energy and have more energy to devote to living the life you want
to lead. Another tool is '10 Daily Habits' and is designed to establish daily routines
that will keep you focused, motivated and appreciative of what you have in your
life. The following exercises are adaptations from part of the Coach U's Personal
Foundation Programme.

Exercise 9.1
What Drains My Energy?

Brainstorming is a technique often used in groups to generate ideas. In this situation I encourage you to brainstorm for yourself and to write down all the thoughts that come into your head in response to the questions posed without censoring them or making a judgement about them. Just record whatever words and thoughts come into your head. You might like to use the table in Figure 9.1 to guide your thoughts.

Resources ◯
◯
◯
◯
◯
●

Tolerations Checklist

All of us are tolerating more than we think. Ask your clients to take a few moments to think about this and complete the following form. The list of tolerations is infinite, different for every person. Try to limit the list to 20-50 tolerations. You would also benefit from this exercise!

What Am I Tolerating?	
Common Tolerations	My Tolerations
Tolerations Areas	1.
Look for tolerations in the following areas (Please note that these a just a few. The list of tolerations is as diverse as people themselves):	2.
	3.
	4.
At Work	5.
Manager	6.
Working Conditions	
Procedures	7.
Requirements	
Hours	8.
Job Tasks	
Environment	9.
Equipment	
Company Culture	10
Co-workers	
Compensation	11.
With Others	12.
Close friends	13.
Spouse	
Children	14.
Social friends	
Relatives	15.
	16
With Yourself	17.
Self-harshness	
Criticism	18.
Behaviors	
Home	19.
Car	
Appearance	20.

© 2003 Coach U. All rights reserved

Figure 9.1   Tolerations checklist

Question 1: Ask yourself 'What work-related activities or situations drain me?'
Take a mental walk through a typical work day from when you arrive until the time you leave.

- Record anything that you react to with irritation, annoyance, a sigh or any other negative response
- Let the words flow to the paper, do not analyse or make judgements about what you write

Question 2: 'What out-of-work related activities or situations drain me?'
Take a mental walk through leaving work and think of some typical activities you do out of work hours.

- Picture yourself travelling and arriving at the place where you live, going in the front door. What do you observe? How do you spend your out-of-work time? What do you do on typical rostered days off work? Are there things on your 'to do' list that you have yet to action?
- Record anything that you react to negatively
- Let the words flow to the paper, do not analyse or make judgements about what you write

Review the list you have compiled. Is there one item on your list you could spend a few minutes on right now, so you can remove it from your list? If so, put this book down, and do it now!

- Notice how your body reacts when you take action and delete something negative or unrewarding from your list
- Can you imagine how you would feel if you removed all these energy draining situations from your life?
- Have you reacted to any items on your list with the thought 'I could not possibly get rid of this. It is too big for me to handle'?
- Are there other items on the list you can easily eliminate? What is stopping you? Do you really want to eliminate them?

If you have been honest in compiling your list, you may experience a reaction that there are some things that you must tolerate in life. But must you? If some items on your list just seem 'too big' or 'too hot to handle' then I recommend that you consider working with a coach, counsellor, career consultant or another healthcare professional to assist you in clarifying what you could do to eliminate the big items on your list. As we explored in Chapter 5 any beliefs you hold about not being able to achieve this can be changed. They are only beliefs, not facts, and you can choose to decide that you are perfectly able to achieve the outcome you desire.

The following client story demonstrates the importance of developing your list, as what Karen may find tedious could be a source of satisfaction for you.

Karen's Story

Karen is 37 and works as the clinical manager for a rehabilitation unit. When she completed this exercise some of the items on her list were:

Work-related things that drain me:

- Files that I haven't got around to filing;
- Having to hunt through piles of reports on my desk to find what I want;
- Staff member who is always late with reports;
- Staff member who takes 30 minutes to tell me something that could take 5 minutes;
- The senior manager who constantly expects me to drop everything I'm doing when they want something;
- The clinician who writes rude emails with copies to other key personnel in the hospital;
- Having to get my manager to sign off items bought that cost more than £••• / $••• yet being responsible for a service budget worth millions!;
- Not finding time for a lunch break because staff constantly want to discuss something with me;
- Hunting for a car park every morning.

Out-of-work things that drain me:

- Car is always dirty;
- Front door needs painting;
- Tap dripping in the kitchen;
- Clothes in the wardrobe that haven't been worn for years;
- 'Wardrobe shrinkage';

- *Friend telephones at inconvenient times;*
- *House not as clean as I want it;*
- *Having to visit an elderly relative every Sunday;*
- *Not having time to do the things I want to do as haven't enough energy;*
- *Going to a regular event I no longer enjoy;*
- *Doing voluntary work every Friday after work.*

When Karen completed this list, she could identify several items that she could do something about immediately. The immediate action she took was

- *Ring the plumber and make an appointment to get the tap fixed.*
- *Place a big plastic bag in her wardrobe in which to put clothes she thought she no longer needed.*
- *Ring a cleaning agency and ask about hourly rates for a house cleaner.*

Next steps:
Reviewing her list, Karen realised that there were some very practical things she could do to reduce situations that drained her. By taking action, making two phone calls and preparing to clean out her wardrobe, she experienced a lift in her energy.

Karen also noticed that some of the activities on her list involved other people's behaviour, which she found challenging, as she did not feel that she had the skills to deal with it.

Karen brought her list to a coaching session to discuss, and developed a strategy to handle these situations. She realised that if she learned assertion skills and understood how to set boundaries she would handle a number of situations in both her professional and personal life more easily.

Karen identified a staff member who had excellent administrative skills. She asked her to establish filing systems and to assist her in managing her files by spending 15 minutes every day filing for her. The staff member reacted very positively to this request, as she gained a sense of satisfaction from establishing new systems. Through recognition and utilisation of a staff member's skill, Karen reduced a stress in her working life.

Reducing activities that you are tolerating allows more time and energy to be spent doing the things you want to do. This may seem straightforward, but often people who have multiple demands made on their time are uncertain how they will spend time if more becomes available. A few minutes invested in doing this exercise could hugely impact on the time you have available in the longer term, as well as the energy levels available to you during that time. The next exercise, 'What energises me?' will assist in incorporating more satisfying and enjoyable activities into your life on a regular basis.

Exercise 9.2
What Energises Me?

This exercise encourages you to create daily habits that are pleasurable for you, and that you look forward to doing. They are not things you 'should' do, but activities that you enjoy doing, that increase your sense of well-being; increase your energy levels or give you a sense of gratitude.

Step 1: Research
Over the next week, take note of things that you do that are enjoyable for you. Keep a record of these activities.

Step 2: Brainstorm
Look at the list you have compiled from Step 1, and write down other activities you could possibly do on a regular basis. You may need to eliminate more time-consuming activities for your weekly or monthly habits list.

Step 3: Develop your '10 Delicious Daily Habits'
(see note, p. 198)
Write down your preferred 10 activities.
These are your d-e-l-i-c-i-o-u-s daily habits! These are habits that may be very simple, only take a few moments, yet enhance your day in some way that is meaningful to you!

It can be helpful in developing your delicious daily habits to make up a chart for the first three months so you can tick off each completed activity each day. Keep the chart in a prominent place to remind you of your intentions. The goal is to complete these activities on at least five out of seven days.

Step 4: Put your '10 Delicious[1] Daily Habits' into action
As you complete your activity, say something positive to reinforce that this is a 'delicious moment'.

Step 5: Review your list as required
I prefer a list for different seasons of the year. Also, refer to Chapter 4, p. 77 and review the eight practical suggestions that assist people in feeling happy. How many of these suggestions can you incorporate into your daily habits?

Some ideas for your 10 delicious daily habits

- Walk for 40 minutes
- Spend quality time with your partner
- Specifically look for someone to praise/acknowledge at work
- Read something you really want to read
- Pause, and look at a beautiful view/picture
- Play with your children
- Walk your dog/stroke your cat
- Read a bed-time story to your children
- Thank the person who cooked your dinner
- Talk with a colleague you respect
- Have coffee with a friend
- Drink water regularly during the day
- Text/email a friend/family member
- Ride your bike for 30 minutes
- Do your favourite floor exercises in front of the TV
- Complete a puzzle/crossword
- Soak in a bath
- Use special soap in the shower
- Meditate for 20 minutes
- Read something that inspires you
- Eat healthy food
- Tell yourself you are gorgeous
- Record in a journal one special thing that happened today
- Have eight hours' sleep

Developing new habits takes time. To assist your progress, I recommend you use a chart similar to the one below (Figure 9.2). Record your 10 Delicious Daily Habits under the activity column, and then tick each day you participate in the activity. Post it in an easily accessible place for the first few weeks to remind you to take time for you! The benefits from this exercise are re-enforced if you say to yourself 'What a delicious moment!' when you have completed the activity. It is said to take 21 days to create a habit, so make sure you do this for at least 21 days for maximum effect.

Resources

10 Daily Habits Chart

Make copies of this chart to keep track of your practice of using 10 Daily Habits.

My 10 Daily Habits								
Week:								
Habit		Day 1	Day 2	Day 3	Day 4	Day 5	Day 6	Day 7
1								
2								
3								
4								
5								
6								
7								
8								
9								
10								

Observations and Notes:

_____

_____

_____

_____

© 2003. Coach U. All rights reserved.

Figure 9.2 10 Daily Habits Chart

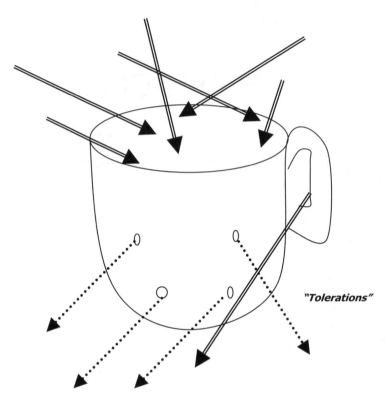

" Delicious Daily Habits"

"Tolerations"

Figure 9.3 Managing energy levels

In managing your energy levels, imagine your energy as water in a cup. As you replenish your energy through activities you enjoy, the level is raised. Activities that drain your energy are like having holes in your cup, the water seeps out, as shown in Figure 9.3.

The goal is to reduce the number of tolerations in your life and therefore close some of the holes in your 'cup'. The more activities you include in your daily life that are important to you and you enjoy, the more energised you can feel.

Once you have the daily habits established in your life, you can start developing '10 Delicious Weekly Habits', '10 Monthly Habits', 10 Annual Habits'! These habits may be based on some of your daily habits but may require more of your time.

For example:

Daily habit: Walk alone for 40 minutes near home or workplace.

Weekly habit: Once a week, walk for 60 minutes near home with a friend or partner.

Monthly: Once a month, walk for 60 minutes in a new environment.

Annually: 10 times a year, walk for 2 hours in a variety of environments.

By identifying activities important to you and ensuring these activities are consciously incorporated into daily living you are beginning to take charge of your energy levels. It is important to write the activities down and acknowledge them when completed, to assist in developing your personalised healthy daily habits.

2. Identifying problems and finding what is causing them

We all face a brick wall from time to time. We can choose to stay in front of it, even bang our head against it. We can sit down and give up or we can turn round and walk away. Or we can get in touch with our inner strength and find ways to climb it, dig under it or navigate round it. We must choose how we deal with a brick wall.

People who work in management will have a number of analytical tools they use to analyse different problems or issues they face at work. However, in my experience, not many use these same tools to analyse a personal problem. At times the problems we face can seem too big to deal with, so having a tool can assist in working through the problem rather than stay living 'in effect' (Chapter 2). One of the most effective ways to overcome these hurdles is to state what the problem is, and then find out all the factors that are contributing to it. By breaking it down into smaller components, and then analysing the factors causing the problem, it becomes more manageable. You might want to consider also using perceptual positioning to help you to see others' perspectives where problems involve others (Chapter 6).

The following tool can be used both personally and professionally and assists in identifying all the factors that are contributing to a problem. It is known by a number of names. The 'Cause & Effect'; 'Ishikawa' or 'Fishbone' diagram (because the diagram looks like a fishbone). It was originally developed by one of the founders of modern management, Kaoru Ishikawa, who introduced quality management into shipyards. Dr W. Edwards Deming adapted the diagram as a useful Total Quality Management tool. My adaptation of the original tool is blended with another management tool, the 'Affinity Diagram', and can be used by an individual or by a group to assist in resolving a common issue.

Exercise 9.3
A Model for Thinking through a Problem

Steps to take to solve a problem using a 'Fishbone' diagram

1. Write down the problem you are facing. Draw a horizontal line across a large piece of paper pointing to the problem.

   e.g. ————————————————————————➤ *The Problem*

2. Write down all the possible causes involved in the problem.

3. Ask yourself:
   Who is involved in this problem?
   What is involved in this problem?
   When does this problem occur?
   Where does this problem occur?
   Why does this problem occur?

Record each cause on a sticky piece of paper and then move the pieces of paper around until you find a natural grouping of responses to which you could attach a label. Each label identifies a key factor causing the problem. The terms 'cause' and 'effect' are used in management material and differ from the same terms used in NLP as discussed in Chapter 2, so we will refer to 'effect' here as the problem, in order to avoid confusion.

Each key factor is drawn as lines off the spine as if they were 'fish bones'.

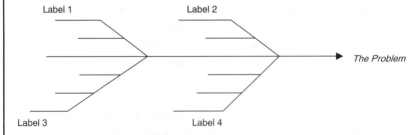

Figure 9.4 Fishbone diagram

All the identified 'causes' are recorded as the smaller lines coming off the 'bones' of the fish

4. Analyse your diagram.
   What does the diagram tell you?
   What areas require further investigation and analysis?
   What could you change immediately?

Sam's Story: Lack of Job Satisfaction

Sam originally trained as a Medical Laboratory Technologist (MLT) and moved into a senior clinical role eight years after qualification. He became the manager of the laboratory and enjoyed this challenging role for a number of years. He came to me for career coaching, as he was no longer getting job satisfaction. I asked Sam what was causing this and he identified the following factors which I wrote up on a whiteboard.

Laboratory equipment breaking down • lack of funding • budget cut-backs • difficulty in finding new qualified staff • poor reports from the auditing agency • lack of support from senior hospital management • paperwork done at weekends • budget proposal rejected by senior manager • feeling tired all the time • equipment replacement programme put on hold • own work PC being used by other people • having to share office with senior clinical MLT • not included in some important discussions being held about the laboratory's future • staff not co-operating with each other

I explained the 'fishbone' diagram, and Sam identified the problem as 'lack of job satisfaction', and items on the list above were the causes. After writing each of the causes on sticky paper, I asked Sam to put them into common themes. He then was asked to label each of the groups. His labels and groups are shown in Figure 9.4.

	Equipment	People	Finance	Management	Personal
CAUSES	▫ laboratory equipment breaking down ▫ equipment replacement programme put on hold ▫ own PC being used by other people	▫ difficulty in finding new qualified staff ▫ staff not co-operating with each other	▫ lack of funding ▫ budget cut-backs ▫ poor reports from the auditing agency	▫ lack of support from senior manage-ment ▫ budget proposal rejected by senior manage-ment ▫ not included in some important discussions being held about the laboratory's future	▫ paperwork done at weekends ▫ feeling tired all the time ▫ having to share office with senior clinical MLT

PROBLEM

Lack of Job Satisfaction

Figure 9.4

> *When Sam saw his responses, he started elaborating on each one and gave me more details of his frustrations. He ended up discussing how he felt about his situation, which shocked him, as he said he normally found it difficult to disclose his feelings. I could hear that his work values were not being met, and I gave him an additional exercise to assist him to understand why he felt out of step with his job.* (See also Values Elicitation in Chapter 5.)

In this case, the 'cause and effect' analytical exercise was used to access how Sam felt about his situation. As an analytical person it provided a safe process for him to talk openly. Sam did leave his job and has made a major career change and is now having his work values met.

The 'Fishbone Diagram' technique allows you to stand back from the obstacle you are facing and use a technique to identify the 'causes' of the 'problem'. Looking at each cause and thinking of all the possible ways to reduce or eliminate that cause is a method to change the 'problem'. You can use the tool in the privacy of your office or as a communication tool for a group wanting to solve a problem.

3. Plan to manage stressful situations

As stated in Chapter 4, figures show that the equivalent of 12.8 million working days a year are lost to stress in the UK alone, with 60% of absences from work due to stress (Health and Safety Executive, 2005). The effects of stress and the implications on our health are well researched and well documented and HSE has identified seven broad categories or the ways in which the workplace potentially contributes to the stress of employees. They include:

- The culture of the organisation. For example, staff involvement in decisions that affect them, and the perception of communication within the workplace.
- The demands of the workplace, such as too much or too little challenge; poor physical environment; exposure to violence, lack of training.
- Relationships and interactions within the workplace, e.g. bullying; low levels of support for the staff.
- How much control the individual has over the tasks they have to perform and whether or not they are included in decision making.
- Coping with change, e.g. managing new technology; restructuring; change in market demands.
- The individual's role, e.g. whether it is ambiguous or if it conflicts with another role.
- The support provided to staff, e.g. matching the person to the job; receiving constructive feedback and advice.

We know a lot about stress. We know that not all stress is bad. Are you able to recognise when you are stressed or identify the triggers that indicate you are about to get stressed?

Acknowledging the possibility that you may experience stress is the first step in recognising it. The next step is to know the signs and symptoms you experience when stressed.

Healthcare professionals are part of the workforce that suffers most from stress, yet not many people turn to them to assist in handling their stress.

So, who is going to help you handle your stress?

This book is about self-empowerment, through which we believe you will professionally develop, so yes, handling the stress starts with you. We need to recognise what we do that works well and do more of it, and recognise what does not work well and do less of it. Coaching can help you to find the difference that makes the difference. We each need to develop a personal range of healthy techniques to respond to stressful situations when they happen, and develop lifestyles that support us. Each person handles stress in different ways, some that are positive and useful and others handle stress by behaving in ways that cause other people increased stress! We encourage you to find a range of techniques that work for you so that you can handle stressful situations more confidently.

> 'Value your own experiences. Learn to ask, "What experiences have I got through in the past that would help and support me in this situation?" Value your own strengths. Learn to ask, "What's needed here? What would make a positive difference? What can I bring to this situation?"'
>
> Stephanie Dowrick (2005)

Develop a personal stress management plan

This can be achieved through four steps.

Step 1: What is your current situation?

The following questions may assist you to analyse your current situation:

* I know I am stressed when . . . (*write as many words or statements to describe how you act and feel when you are stressed*).

* I know I am NOT stressed when . . . (*write as many words or statements to describe how you act and feel when you are not stressed*).

* Techniques that I have used to handle a stressful situation include . . . (*write down as many techniques that you can think of that you have used effectively*).

* Techniques that assisted me most in feeling less stressed are. . . . (*circle the techniques that were positive for you*).

- Other techniques I have heard of but have not tried are . . . (*record any you have heard or read about*)

- Which of these am I prepared to find out more about and use to assess their effectiveness for me in a stressful situation?. . . . (*circle the techniques you are prepared to try*)

- Do I need more information or assistance in developing a personal stress management plan? . . . (*Yes/No. Record the information you require and/or who could assist you develop your plan*)

- When will I write my Personal Stress Management Plan? (*put down a date that is realistic and that you are genuinely prepared to honour*)

Once you have this information about your current way of handling stress, it is important that you take action! Taking action is one of the best ways of regaining a sense of control over feeling stressed, along with developing your own personal stress management plan.

Step 2: What are the options you could consider?

The five key areas to consider are:

1. Physical activity: 20 minutes of aerobic activity three times a week is a common minimum recommendation
2. Nutrition: Eat well and be guided by the food guide pyramid (www.ext. nodak.edu/extpubs/yf/foods/he509-1.gif)
3. Attitude: Think positively and reduce negative thoughts
4. Social support: Develop positive networks
5. Relaxation: Develop a relaxation technique that works for you; take time for your hobbies

Review each of the five areas, and consider all the options available to you. If you already have techniques that work for you, write them in your plan to acknowledge the important positive role these activities have in supporting you already.

Complete your choices and record them in your personal chart.

Step 3: Write up your plan

Review your chart and assess what is realistic for you to add into your daily, weekly or monthly routine. How many of the stress management techniques can be part of your '10 Delicious Daily Habits' mentioned earlier in this chapter?

Step 4: Act on your plan

If you find that you do not put your plan into action, for what ever reason, then you are reducing your opportunity to have control in the way you live your life and the results you allow yourself to achieve. Are you going to wait for a critical incident' (Chapter 4) to occur in your life before you take care of your needs? If you find you are putting your needs 'on hold', then a coach could assist you in developing and implementing your plan.

Here is an example of a stress management plan developed by a client. New activities she introduced are in italics

Area	Activity	Frequency		
		Daily	Weekly	Monthly
Physical	20 minutes walk with partner	√		
	Dancing to rock'n'roll music	√		
	Gardening		√	
Nutrition	*Sit at the table when I eat*	√		
	Drink 6 glasses water	√		
	Eat fruit mid-morning & afternoon	√		
	Eat vegetables from our garden	√		
	Enjoy home-made wholegrain cereal	√		
Attitude	*Record 3 things I am grateful about today in my journal each evening*	√		
	Discuss progress with coach			√
	Using 'I' statements when discussing issues at work (being at cause – pp. 14 and 20)	√		
	'STOP', and rephrase when I hear myself talking negatively about me! (see section on reframing p. 108)	√		
Social Support	Spending quality time with my partner	√		
	Time with supportive colleague at work		√	
	Playing bridge		√	
	Meeting with family members			√
Relaxation	Walk around my garden	√		
	Write in my journal	√		
	Listen to classical music		√	
	Learn a new relaxation technique			
	Have a bath before bed	√		

The plan is simple, personalised and most importantly thought about at a conscious level. This client started her day quietly writing in her journal, and then went to a private part of her home and turned on the rock 'n roll music and danced slowly at first and gradually built up to have an aerobic workout. She loved this new way of starting her day, and it set her in a positive frame of mind which was one of her major challenges. During the day, if she became upset or stressed about something at work she got up and went for a five-minute walk to reduce her agitation. In the evening, she gradually reduced the activity levels. She would spend time with her partner while they walked around their beautiful garden discussing their day and their children's activities. She then wrote three positive things about her day in her journal before having a bath while she listened to classical music. By bed-time she was feeling relaxed and ready for a good sleep. These simple changes in her daily life enhanced her quality of life tremendously, and she found she handled stressful situations more easily.

Techniques for handling stress

Three techniques that we find effective for handling stressful situations are:

1. Mental rehearsal and positive internal dialogue.
2. The HeartMath Appreciation® Technique.
3. Immediate stress diffuser techniques.

1. *Mental rehearsal and positive internal dialogue*

Chapter 2 introduced a Communication Model that highlights our internal communication processes, which in turn impact on our behaviours, actions and results. The power of our internal dialogue, our self talk or internal voice, can often be an obstacle because that voice can be our harshest critic. However, our self talk can be used to assist us if we find ways to use its power in a positive way.

Mental rehearsal or visualisation is a tool that has been used by many, including athletes and sports people to improve their performance (see Chapter 8 for use of mental rehearsal in self-management). If you can picture a scene, no matter how hazy the picture may be, this technique could be a helpful one for you to manage situations that you find stressful or in which you want to improve your performance. Visualisation is not easy for everyone at first as we each process information in our preferred and natural way. However, with practice everyone can learn to do it better and more easily.

This mental rehearsal technique could be used in a range of situations that healthcare professionals face such as:

- telling patients and their families about poor test results
- performing a challenging technique
- resuscitating patients
- presenting a paper at a conference
- sitting an examination
- going for a job interview
- speaking in public or to the media
- discussing a difficult subject with a staff member
- presenting a new idea at a staff meeting
- facilitating a staff meeting
- tutoring a new group of students

Exercise 9.4
Mental Rehearsal (2)

The five steps required in mental rehearsal with positive internal dialogue are:

1. Identify a situation that you want to improve.

2. Find a quiet place where you will not be disturbed, and think about the specific changes you want to make. Think about how you want the situation to be (not how you don't want it to be). Take note of how you want to act and feel in the situation. Make it as sensory, rich and compelling as possible. What will it sound like? What will you be saying? How will you feel? What will you be doing? It may be helpful to write out the scenario first. Every action is positive, confident, and assists in developing how you want to be in this situation. We know that we will get what we focus on, so we need to focus on what we want.

3. Once you have a clear picture of what you want, sit or lie in a comfortable position, close your eyes and breathe slowly. Be aware of your breathing. Take three or four deep breaths concentrating on breathing out any feelings of concern or doubt you may have. As you breathe in concentrate on what you want more of, such as being positive and confident. Continue to breathe in confidence and positivity and exhale concerns.

4. See yourself in the situation you want to improve, and rehearse the mental picture you have made with positive self-talk to support your actions. Observe how you are behaving in the situation and how you

are feeling. See your desired outcome and say to yourself whatever you need to hear to make this possible. For example, 'I am relaxed and confident'. 'I am in control of my emotions and I can do this'. 'I am achieving my desired goal'. Trust yourself. You know what you need to say to make this easy to do. Make your words very positive, strong and supportive and talk to yourself in the present tense, as if you were actually in the situation and acting and feeling in the desired way.

5. Repeat the mental rehearsal regularly or as part of your preparation for a specific event.

This technique does not take a lot of time, and with practice can be used easily for a number of situations. It may only take a few minutes in bed each night for three or four days before the actual event, as Victoria's story below illustrates.

Victoria's Story

Victoria is a registrar who has to give her first major presentation at an international conference. She has confidence in the research she has done, and has developed excellent visuals to support her presentation. Her main issue is how nervous she feels before presenting in front of an audience, especially to colleagues and people she really respects. On the day of giving a presentation, she feels ill, cannot eat and has to really talk herself into attending the seminar. She very much wants to present at this particular conference, and sought assistance with handling her fear of public speaking.

As her coach, I soon discovered that Victoria had the ability to visualise what her presentation would be like. However, the picture she created in her head focused on every possible situation that could go wrong. She saw herself forgetting her notes, tripping on the steps, having a coughing attack and the PowerPoint presentation failing her. No wonder she felt so nervous!

I asked Victoria to visualise a new picture for this situation, to include as much detail as possible, and with an accompanying audio clip. Some of the things that Victoria included in her new clip were:

- *Showering with her favourite soap on the morning of the presentation, telling herself that she is feeling calm, confident and capable.*

- *Looking in the mirror, giving herself a big 'thumbs up' sign and the biggest smile possible and saying 'Wow, you are so good at presenting papers! You are so calm, confident and capable and can handle any situation'.*

- *Eating breakfast, she has her favourite cereal, a piece of fruit and a cup of coffee. She tells herself that this food is fuelling her brain so that she is attentive, alert and able to handle any situation that arises.*

- *Selecting the clothes that she will wear for the presentation, she puts each garment on and tells herself that she is feeling very calm, very confident and very capable. She reassures herself that she has done the research and that she is the expert in her chosen topic.*

- *Arriving at the venue for the presentation, Victoria allows time to find the correct conference room, and as she enters the room she feels calmness enveloping her.*

- *Walking to the front of the conference room she takes in slow deep breaths and says that she is feeling calm, confident and capable.*

- *Victoria has her papers ready. The audio-visuals are ready. She sees herself taking the time, not rushing and looking very confident. She then looks at her audience, takes in a deep breath, smiles and introduces her presentation.*

- *Ending the presentation, Victoria feels very calm and focused. She answers several questions confidently and then calmly gathers her notes and walks away from the centre of attention and hears the applause as she returns to her seat. She is feeling very calm, confident and capable.*

- *The week before the presentation, Victoria mentally rehearsed her script every day before she went to sleep. She found that on the actual day, she was living the script she had written. She did forget to have her favourite soap available but she said that she repeated the phrase 'I am calm, confident and capable and can handle whatever comes my way', and did not let this detail upset her. She reported a sense of calmness as she was being introduced and as she stepped forward and placed her papers on the rostrum.*

Victoria was delighted by how this technique helped her, and planned to use it for other situations she faced in life.

The main points in the mental rehearsal process are:

- To make your picture in the present, as if the event is happening now.
- Perform the actions with confidence.
- Develop some key words of support in the script. Victoria's phrase was 'calm, confident and capable'.

The use of anchoring, described in Chapter 8, alongside mental rehearsal would be a simple way to further enhance the effectiveness of this technique.

2. The HeartMath Appreciation® Technique

The Institute of HeartMath® (see note, p. 198) has conducted research for more than 15 years on the physiology of and relationship between the heart, stress and emotions. Their research has been published in journals such as *American Journal of Cardiology*, *Stress Medicine* and *Preventive Cardiology*. HeartMath researchers have found that measuring our changing heart rhythms (heart rate variability) gives a consistent reflection of our internal stress and emotional state. When the heart rate variability is measured in a person who is feeling calm and confident, the smooth, rolling hills-like pattern produced in the heart rate variability graph is said to be in 'coherence'. When the heart rate variability is measured in a person who is upset, stressed or angry the chaotic pattern produced is called 'incoherence'.

The Institute's extensive research concludes that sincere, positive feelings boost the immune system while negative emotions may suppress the immune response for up to six hours after the emotional response to an event; and the risk of developing heart disease is significantly increased for people who impulsively vent their anger as well as those who tend to repress their feelings. The results of this research alone could be enough for most of us to want to develop an effective way of managing our emotional response to stressful situations.

Based on their research, the Institute of HeartMath has developed a number of scientifically validated tools and technologies that assist people in sustaining positive emotions and physiological coherence, thereby reducing stress. There are a number of HeartMath tools that I use, and which have also been of benefit to many of my clients. One simple exercise I can give you now to get you started is good to practise at any time of the day to help you get into coherence. Also, it feels great!

Exercise 8.5
Appreciation Exercise

Take short, one- or two-minute, appreciation breaks during the day. Breathe deeply through the area of the heart, four to five seconds in and then four to five seconds out. While doing so, try and hold a feeling of appreciation in the area of your heart. It can be a feeling of appreciation for a partner, child, friend, your pet, a favorite place, a fun holiday, etc. The key is to hold a sincere feeling towards something, not just to have a mental image. Some people find it helps to use a photo of someone that they care for and appreciate to help them activate a genuine heart feeling of appreciation.

The genuine heart feeling of appreciation helps to build heart coherence so that when we are faced with challenging situations, we have an accumulation of calm, balance and clarity. The exercise of activating a positive feeling like appreciation literally shifts our physiology, helping to balance our heart rhythms and nervous system, and creates more coherence between the heart, brain and the rest of the body. (Based on HeartMath research published in *American Journal of Cardiology*, 1995.)

This simple exercise can be used at any time as a quick and effective way to rebalance your emotions. You do not have to wait for a stressful situation to practise this; I encourage you to use it regularly during the day. If you are interested in the research papers, abstracts and reports that have been written in peer reviewed journals I encourage you to view the website www.heartmath.org.

3. Immediate stress defusing techniques

Before we respond we make a choice. In that split second we have incredible power to decide which way to go. If we can elongate that time, even by a fleeting moment, we give ourselves the opportunity to grow and develop. Maybe for some it would be enough even to recognise that there is a momentary pause in which you make those huge decisions about how to respond.

Your stress management plan needs to include techniques that assist you the minute you recognise you are under stress. Your body will be telling you that it has received a trigger, and as a result may also be about to set up a negative anchor in response, and you need to develop the ability to listen to the signals so you can intervene as soon as possible. When you recognise a trigger, pause before you respond, so that you can choose your response. By recognising the trigger and using this knowledge, you can immediately initiate the stress management technique that works best for you and therefore have even more control over stressful events in life. There are many things in life over which we have no direct influence but there is one aspect in life that we do have control of, and that is how we respond to situations we face. We may wish to change other people's behaviour, but the only behaviour we can really change is our own (Review Chapter 2: Self-Empowerment). We cannot change their actions, and we can change our reactions. We encourage you to take responsibility for things that you can influence, starting with how you choose to respond to a situation you find stressful.

The following four scenarios are offered to stimulate your imagination and give you ideas for developing a range of techniques that work for you.

- The senior nurse has just made sarcastic comments to you in front of a group of other staff. You are furious but do not want to react to the situation. You go to the nearest linen room and shut the door. You take in a deep breath and let out a 'silent' scream that no-one can hear. You take in another deep breath and emit another 'silent scream'. You then take in three slow deep breaths and breathe them out slowly telling yourself that you handled the comments with dignity. You then let out any negative feelings that remain. You return to work knowing that the comments have said more about the senior nurse than they have about you.

- The report is due in today. You have 30 minutes' uninterrupted time at your computer when you notice the tension in your shoulders. You immediately drop your shoulders, stop typing and slowly turn your head to the right and slowly to the left. You take in a deep breath through your nose and let your stomach expand. You breathe out slowly and drop your shoulders. You shut your office door and turn off the phone and so take practical steps to reduce disturbances and therefore create the environment to get your work done. You continue with your report.

- You have just been part of the team in the Emergency Department assisting the victims of a road crash. Your part is finished, and you performed your role well. However, you notice a knot in your stomach as you leave. You look at your hands, and they are shaking slightly and you feel tears well up. As you walk to your changing room, you take in a deep breath and picture the beautiful beach you discovered on your last holiday. It feels warm, pretty and the water looks cool. You imagine this picture is wrapped around your heart, and you take in another deep breath. As you enter the changing room a colleague asks you how your day is going. You ask them if they have a moment ot two to spare as you want to have a cup of tea and a talk about what you have been doing during the last three hours.

- You have had a demanding day at work including five staff coming to you about an incident that has upset them. It involves three other staff members, but none of them was available for you to interview that day so you could find out their version of the incident. You have booked times with them for the next day. However the issues are going round and round in your head. As you are driving home alone, you feel the anger and frustration building up inside. You close the car windows and turn up the radio to drown your screams of frustration. You feel the physical tension subsiding; however later in the evening your thoughts are still focused on your concerns and fears about the described incident. You find a large piece of paper and write down all the thoughts running through your head. You do not censor your thoughts and feelings and just write and write and write until no more words flow onto the page. You are feeling calm and very tired, and before you go to bed you shred everything you have written as you do not want anyone else to read what thoughts had been in your head.

Developing stress diffusing techniques that work for you is very empowering. As you become more familiar with what causes you stress, and how your body reacts to stress, you will learn how to respond healthily to stressful situations instead of reacting unhealthily. Unhealthy reactions, such as denial that you experience stress or attempting to block your reactions through the use of alcohol or drugs, are going to create many more obstacles in your future life.

This whole process of reaction links very well to the NLP cause and effect model outlined in Chapter 2, which describes taking responsibility for yourself, rather than blaming others or environmental factors. It also reaffirms the close mind-body link as well as demonstrating practical ways in which you can use the Communication Model to alter your state and physiology to impact on the Internal Representations you hold about a situation. By understanding how these processes work, we give ourselves an awareness of that vital space before we react, so that we can choose our reaction to get the results we want.

Maintaining momentum

Another common obstacle for people is implementing and maintaining the stages of a plan. Enthusiasm, good intentions and a new year are all helpful in the planning stage, but we need more than good intentions to carry out our plans. If you do tend to start new plans and soon run out of energy for them, having a buddy or a coach could help. The fact that we have someone else who knows about our plan and that we arrange to see them or call them on a regular basis can assist many people in overcoming procrastination or running out of enthusiasm. Using time lines effectively (Chapter 8) can also help to prevent procrastination by ensuring you are continually drawn forward to your future goals.

Have you ever considered finding yourself a coach? A coach does not tell you what to do or how to live your life. A coach is there to assist you discover how you want your life to be and what steps you can take to make that dream a reality. You may get challenged by your coach; however, you will know that you have this person who is giving you encouragement and exercises to assist you in finding your own answers to your questions in life. Your coach may be the only person who is interested in all of your roles in life and what you want from them. Your coach will listen to you, and will be your confidant outside of your family, friends and colleagues and who can often hold the 'bigger picture' for you. A good coach will also have at their disposal a range of tools and techniques to help you to get the results you want.

In order to ensure you work with someone who is qualified to give a recognised level of coaching service, ensure that you look for recognised credentials when forming a new coaching relationship. At the end of the next chapter there are some notes on coaching accreditation and some ideas on how to find a qualified coach.

Summary

This chapter has been about finding a way around obstacles that we have commonly encountered with our work as healthcare professionals. The goal is to encourage you to find solutions to issues that may have in the past prevented you performing your professional role in the way that you really wanted to. Having methods for managing your energy levels; identifying problems and what is causing them, and developing your personalised stress management plan will not only enhance your professional life, but it will also flow over into your non-work life. You will feel more in control and your increased sense of enjoyment will be noticed and appreciated by those with whom you come into contact. People will notice a positive change in you, and may be curious as to what you have done to make that change. You could cause a positive ripple effect as a role model for others, which in turn could hugely impact on the level of patient care given to those seeking your advice. And it all started with you committing to make positive changes in your life and by reading this book! Can you imagine how different your life would be if you had the techniques to ensure you reached all the goals you set, how empowered you would feel? Can you imagine how much more you would achieve? You now have everything you need to make this a reality and we hope you make the most of it and enjoy every minute of putting it into practice and living your dreams.

References

Dowrick, S. (2005) *Choose Happiness: Life & soul essentials.* London, Allen & Unwin.
Health and Safety Executive (2005) *Survey of Self-reported Work-related Illness* (SWI04/05).

Notes

Coach U, founded in 1988. is the largest provider of online training for people entering the professional field of personal training. www.coachinc.com

10 Daily Habits is a Coach U tool which has been adapted by Fiona Miller to '10 Delicious Daily Habits'. Fiona is a master NLP practitioner and ICF certified professional coach from Scotland, currently residing in New Zealand.

Institute of HeartMath® 14700 West Park Avenue, Boulder Creek, California, USA www.heartmath.org

A few final thoughts

10

Suzanne Henwood

What is it you now believe? About yourself? About your future? It is those beliefs that will determine your final pathway to success. Acknowledging and using the power that lies within you can be exactly what you want to be.

This book is about self-empowerment, it is all about you, about identifying and creating the life you want to live, both in work and at home. It is our belief that it is through true self-empowerment that you will achieve effective personal and professional development. Our aim in writing this book has been to share with you a set of tools which we have found to be effective in our own lives and in our own work as coaches and trainers in healthcare. We have brought those tools together within a framework for self-empowerment, a framework which, if you follow it from start to finish, will enable you to easily and successfully make the changes you want to make, so that you can achieve even more of the results you want to achieve. We hope that in addition you will share what you have learnt with your colleagues, and that, together, you will create a lasting impact on the quality of patient care within your own field of health service practice.

The only person who can hold you back is you. Believe in your own ability to make the changes and believe in your ability to create your future and you will be amazed at how easily you can make the changes you want to make. If you are not yet at the point where you can accept this statement, we would urge you to find a coach and to do whatever it is that you need to do to get to that point in your own personal journey. It is not a weakness to accept help, indeed it is a sign of a strong and healthy mind that will reach out and look for ways to be even more effective. Don't let anything hold you back: this is your chance to be who you want to be.

It is our belief that to work in healthcare is a privilege and an honour. To be allowed to get alongside those who are at times vulnerable and afraid, and to be given the opportunity to make a difference for them through the quality of service we provide and the skills we can offer, is both a responsibility and an enormous honour. We hope that by understanding yourself in more depth and taking the steps to empower yourself and care for and value yourselves, you will be even more effective carers and leaders in your field, and that you will use what you have learnt here and apply it in your own workplace in a way that works for you, your team and your patients. Mahatma Gandhi said: 'We must become the change we want to see': that change starts with us and grows from there. So who is it you want to be at work and at home and what changes are you already putting in place to make that a reality?

We started this book by getting you to focus on yourself and we want to end it the same way. You will already have noticed positive changes inside as you worked through the tools outlined in this book and we would encourage you to keep using the tools over and over as you grow and learn more about yourself. Maybe you could consider using a personal development diary to record those changes over time, to highlight just how effective the tools have been. Remember that many of these tools can be found on our website at www.wiley.com/go/nlphealthcare so that you can revisit them as often as you like. Use the code indicated at www.wiley.com/go/nlphealthcare to gain access.

You can use many of the tools here as a framework to help you to record your development, so consider integrating them into your professional CPD requirements. We would urge you to resist the temptation just to collect CPD hours or points, as this does nothing to demonstrate real development. Instead you can use the framework here to genuinely reflect on and evaluate the changes in yourself and the quality of the service you offer as a result of your development activities, by analysing the effect on you and your practice.

As you have worked through the book, you will have explored areas in your life in new ways and you may have found some areas that you wish to explore in greater depth. If you have never considered using a coach or an independent clinical supervisor you might like to take that step to further consolidate what you have learned about yourself while reading this book. There are many coaches and styles of coaching out there and we would urge you to ensure that you select one who has a respected qualification and accepted credentials to ensure that you get the maximum benefit from your investment. At the end of this chapter we give some suggestions of accreditations you might like to look for to give you some assurance of quality in coaching practice. In the future it is likely that some form of regulation will be brought in to coaching to assure quality. Until then you should ask around, find a coach who you know of, or who has been recommended to you, who has demonstrated their effectiveness with someone you know. Failing that, ask the associations who work to introduce standards to recommend a coach in your area.

We also include a 'recommended reading' section at the end of the book which outlines some of our favourite books. This list is not in any way exhaustive; it merely represents books we have read and enjoyed and which have taught us things which relate to the topics we have covered here. We hope you will use these suggestions to explore many of the concepts we have introduced in greater depth. We also offer a range of coaching and training opportunities, and you will find our contact details at the end of this chapter should you want to explore any additional learning with us. For example we have set up, through Henwood Associates (South East) Ltd, the first ever NLP Diploma for Healthcare Professionals, a project which we are really excited about in terms of taking the ideas in this book, and much more, out into the healthcare environment, so it can really start to have an impact. Or maybe you are already considering some more formal NLP or coaching qualification. Again, as with coaching, take advice and ensure you train with people who care about the standards of those they certificate, train with those who will not certificate people who they do not think are competent to practise. The trainers we have worked with ourselves are also listed at the end of this book to give you some guidance. For example, if training is done in large groups you might want to ask specifically how your competence to use the tools taught will be assessed so you can be confident in your own ability, before using them in practice.

As a result of reading this book you will have already started to think about, and to create, your future. We hope that you are now dreaming dreams of all that you want to achieve and all that you want to be in your life. It is well accepted in management and leadership circles that those who are high achievers are those who have a clear vision of where it is they are going. If you have used the tools in this book, you now have a vision and a clear set of goals to work towards and a life purpose to fulfil; you can start living your dreams. As you achieve your goals and set new ones do share your success with us and with your colleagues; we would love to hear what a difference this book has made to you and your patients.

We hope that we have sparked in you a renewed passion for your chosen profession and for your patients, a new energy and a different way of working and thinking. We hope that through this book you will find renewed satisfaction and success in your workplace, either the same workplace or in pastures new. We have reached out to you from the pages of this book and we ask you to take seriously your own future, to invest in yourself and to set yourself up for success. We have personally experienced the massive change which is possible through using these techniques. It is our desire to share them with you and to offer you the same opportunity to change your life, in the way you want to change it, be that a big change or small change, so that you get the results you want to get. We know the changes outlined in the stories in this book are available to you too and we hope you have embraced the tools with sincerity and commitment and that you are already starting to reap the rewards.

We wish you futures where your dreams are fulfilled and where the areas beyond your dreams become reality. Marianne Williamson said:

> *Our deepest fear is not that we are inadequate. Our deepest fear is that we are powerful beyond measure. It is our light, not our darkness that most frightens us. We ask ourselves, who am I to be brilliant, gorgeous, talented and fabulous? Actually, who are you not to be? You are a child of God. Your playing small doesn't serve the world. There is nothing enlightening about shrinking so that other people won't feel insecure around you*

Be who you want to be: live life to the full: be true to your inner self – and just as importantly, have fun! If you compromise yourself and compromise what it is you want to achieve you are unlikely to find satisfaction or happiness in work or in life generally. Connect with your inner self, recognise your true worth and let others see just how amazing you are.

Suzanne Henwood (www.henwoodassociates.co.uk)
Jim Lister (www.changepartnership.co.uk)
Liz Holland (www.lizholland.biz)

Reference

Williamson, M. (1992) *A Return to Love: Reflections on the principles of a course in miracles.* London, HarperCollins.

Appendix

NLP training

There are many excellent NLP trainers available. It is impossible to mention them all here and in no way are we suggesting that any not mentioned below should not be on the list. What we can do here is recommend those of whom we have personal knowledge, who we know are passionate about the standards of those qualifying with them and who in the UK aim to establish standards for all to follow. We recommend here the people who trained us and to whom we are indebted for their expertise in passing on their knowledge in a way that has transferred that passion about the potential of NLP to transform lives.

If you are considering training in NLP at practitioner or master practitioner level you might like to consider contacting:

Jeremy Lazarus of The Lazarus Consultancy (www.thelazarus.com)

Lisa Wake of Awaken Consulting (www.awakenconsulting.co.uk)

John Seymour Associates (www.john-seymour-associates.co.uk)

You can also look for trainer accreditation status at associations such as ANLP (www.anlp.org) for guidance on those who have sought specific accreditation for NLP training.

For details regarding the NLP Diploma for Healthcare Professionals, see www.henwoodassociates.co.uk.

Coaching accreditation

While this list is not exhaustive, it includes those organisations of whom we have personal experience and which may be useful to consult when looking for an accredited coach:

- ANLP (www.anlp.org) The Association of NLP holds a list of NLP qualified coaches and is working hard to establish national standards for NLP practice and ongoing competence through CPD.
- Association for Coaching (www.associationforcoaching.com) ensures that its members are suitably qualified as coaches. Different levels of membership indicate the range of experience a coach has.

- International Coach Federation (www.coachfederation.org/ICF/) Members have to undergo an accreditation process to confirm the standard of their training, as well as demonstrating that they are experienced practitioners.

- Coach U (www.coachu.com and www.findacoach.com/index.html) Coach U offers training programmes and an index of their international coaches. Coach U programmes are accredited by the International Coach Federation.

Reading list

This list is not exhaustive and represents books we have read and enjoyed and which have helped us to extend our understanding of the concepts outlined in this book. They are listed alphabetically and not in any order of preference.

Beliefs: Pathways to Health and Well Being

Robert Dilts, Tim Hallbom and Suzi Smith (1990) Metamorphous Press, Portland, Oregon, USA

This is a great book for exploring in greater depth the issue of belief change. It offers the 'how to' of belief change work and also cites actual case consultations of the tools in use.

Choose Happiness: Life & Soul Essentials

Stephanie Dowrick (2005) Allen & Unwin, London

Stephanie Dowrick was born in New Zealand and lived in London for many years. She founded the independent publishing house The Women's Press. In 1983 she moved to Australia where she still lives. Having lived in different places, been a psychotherapist, publisher, writer and Interfaith Minister she brings an eclectic background to her writing. *Choose Happiness* is a book that can be read from front to back, or dipped into at any point. It is a practical and universal book and one we enjoy having to hand. Chapter headings include: Trust who you are; Let your values and goals work for you; Choose your attitudes and responses; Build self-respect; Consider others; Honour the people you love; Think and act positively.

Co-active Coaching

Laura Whitworth, Henry Kimsey-House, Phil Sandahl (1998) Davies-Black Publishing

This is one of the earlier coaching books, yet is still relevant today. If you are interested in coaching others and want to develop your skills, this is a very readable and practical book. It has coaching session dialogues, and a toolkit.

Coach Yourself to Success

Talane Miedaner (2000) Contemporary Books a division of TC/ Contemporary Publishing Group Inc.

Talene is a Coach U graduate from America who now lives with her family in the UK. This is a self-help book with 101 tips to assist people in reaching their personal and professional objectives. Her tips are based on the Coach U training programme and it can be used for looking at specific areas you want to improve, or you can go through the exercises in the order they are set out.

Excuse Me, Your Life is Waiting: the astonishing power of positive feelings

Lynn Grabhorn (2000) Hodder and Stoughton, London

If you want to look in greater depth at the concept of 'You get what you focus on' this is the book for you. It is a very easy read and gives lots of advice about how to change your life through the power of your thinking.

Flying Start: Coaching your children for life

Emma Sargent (2006) Cyan and Marshall Cavendish Editions, London

This is an excellent book, written without jargon and completely accessible to people who are not trained in NLP. It offers many of the tools in a format suitable for children and while it is written for parents it would be equally suitable for use with paediatric patients where you have the opportunity to work with the child over a period of time and build a relationship with them to make their experiences of healthcare less traumatic.

Molecules of Emotion: Why you feel the way you feel

Candace B Pert (1997) Simon and Schuster, London

For those readers who want to explore the evidence for the biomolecular basis of our emotions, this is the book for you. If you want to look more at how NLP and other associated techniques work, this is worth a read. It provides evidence for the mind-body link in a very readable form.

NLP at Work: The difference that makes a difference in business

Sue Knight (2002, 2nd Edition) Nicholas Brearley Publishing, London

This is one of the most easy to read handbooks of NLP that we have found.

While it is written for a business context, it is still useful for those working in healthcare. If you want a good basic description of what NLP is, this book outlines it for you in Chapter 1. It then goes on to present many of the NLP tools in a very user-friendly way. You could then apply these tools to your own work context.

Neuro-Linguistic Programming for Dummies

Romilla Ready and Kate Burton (2004) John Wiley & Sons Ltd, Chichester

As you would expect from a 'For Dummies' series this is a very accessible book about NLP and includes a little bit of work on time lines. It is very easy to read and offers useful tips and practical exercises throughout. Again, you could then apply these tools to your own work context.

The 7 Habits of Highly Effective People

Stephen R. Covey (1990) Simon and Schuster, New York

This book has been available for a long time, and can be considered a classic management book. It has been translated into more than 35 languages and it is still a good starting place for people who are interested in the difference between 'management' and 'leadership'.

The 8th Habit

Stephen R Covey (2004) Simon and Schuster, London

This new addition to the 7 Habits of Highly Effective People is an easy read and fits very easily alongside NLP philosophy. In particular it is interesting to look at the notion of the legacy you will leave behind. The book explores people's 'profound yearning' to find their 'true voice, to matter, to make a difference, to find greatness'.

The Structure of Magic (Volumes I and II)

Richard Bandler and John Grinder (1975 and 1976) Science and Behavior Books Inc, Palo Alto, California

In any reading list on NLP we have to include these, as this is where it all began.

Words that Change Minds: Mastering the language of influence

Shelle Rose Charvet (1997, 2nd Edition) Kendall/Hunt Publishing Company, Dubuque, Iowa

This is a book which looks in greater depth at the power of language. It looks at the language someone uses and predicts from that how they will behave in certain situations. It also looks at how you can select language deliberately to influence others.

Websites

www.ANLP.org

This is a great site to pick up tips about NLP. It will also help you find an NLP practitioner in your area. You can use it to find accredited NLP trainers and to find lots of useful resources around the subject.

www.coachfederation.org/ICF/

One way to find a coach who belongs to a professional coaching organisation is to contact the International Coach Federation (ICF) which has more than 10,000 coach members in 80 countries. To attain full membership of the ICF coaches have to go through an accreditation process to ensure that their training is of a high standard and that they are experienced practitioners.

www.coachu.com & www.findacoach.com/index.html

Coach U offers training programmes and an index of their international coaches. Coach U training programmes have been offered since 1992, and they are accredited by the International Coach Federation. This 'virtual university' teaches through teleclasses, so students come from all parts of the world which adds a positive dimension to the classes. It is a practical, experiential programme for people who learn best by doing. There are also coach training events offered in person (e.g. Core Essentials Fast Track Programme) in North America, Europe, Australia, New Zealand and Singapore. Coach U offers free introductory teleclasses so you can assess whether this training programme suits your style of learning.

www.heartmath.org

If you have an interest in reducing stress, this is a very useful website. The Institute of HeartMath conducts research to develop scientifically validated, practical tools that enable people to improve their health and quality of life. Their research includes emotional physiology and heart-brain interactions, clinical studies and physiology of learning and performance. Their website offers interesting reading material, access to a free newsletter and daily 'heart quotes', plus specific sites for health professionals. Access to some parts of the site requires membership. They also sell products and training programmes though the site.

www.mindtools.com

This is an excellent site for a range of tools to assist people in the workplace. Time management, stress management, leadership, problem solving and decision making tools are all included. Their e-letter keeps you up to date with their tools. Some are classic and well known and others new and worth experimenting with.

www.nlpweekly.com

Another site which offers a useful free newsletter which provides tips and discussion pieces around NLP techniques.

www.reflectivehappiness.com

Positive Psychology. Dr Martin Seligman developed a programme which accurately measured and improved depression and happiness in over 90% of test subjects. You can take assessments to find out your Authentic Happiness Index; your place on the CES-D scale, assessing your depression index during the past week, and your VIA Signature Strengths. The first month is free, after which there is a small monthly fee. Each month there are questions answered by Dr Seligman, a new exercise to increase your happiness, and positive psychology booklists. Positive Psychology may not yet be a highly respected research area, but we suggest taking a look and completing some of the exercises in order to make up your own mind.

www.saladltd.co.uk
This is a great site for resources relating to NLP, and Jamie Smart offers a free newsletter and a free email happiness tip to keep you boosted each week.

http://www.sueknight.co.uk/Publications/articlesindex.htm
This is a great page from which to pick up some articles written by Sue Knight, the author of *NLP At Work*.

List of exercises

2.1   Putting Yourself at Cause
2.2   Understanding Communication
2.3   Becoming Aware of Our World
2.4   Hearing Internal Dialogue
2.5   Working at Cause

3.1   Building Rapport
3.2   Working with Eye Patterns

4.1   Wheel of Life
4.2   Begin with the End in Mind
4.3   CCCSS Model

5.1   Exploring your Beliefs
5.2   Eliciting Values at Work
5.3   Logical Levels of Change

6.1   Getting to the Meaning
6.2   Exploring Perception Gaps
6.3   Reframing
6.4   Perceptual Positioning

7.1   Finding My Life's Purpose
7.2   Taking Charge of My Thought Processes
7.3   Goal Setting
7.4   Self Coaching Discussion

Index